USMLE
Step 1

Integrated
Vignettes

© 2019 Kaplan Publishing

Published by Kaplan Publishing, a division of Kaplan, Inc.
750 Third Avenue
New York, NY 10017

Printed in the United States of America

10 9 8 7 6 5 4 3 2 1

ISBN-13: 978-1-5062-4690-1

Kaplan Publishing books are available at special quantity discounts to use for sales promotions, employee premiums, or educational purposes. For more information or to order books, please call the Simon & Schuster special sales department at 866-506-1949.

Lead Editor

Heather Farmer Hoffmann, MD
Adjunct Assistant Professor of Public Health
Franklin & Marshall College
Lancaster, PA

We want to hear what you think. What do you like or not like about the book?

Please email us at **medfeedback@kaplan.com**.

Table of Contents

How to Use This Book

In preparation for the practice of medicine, medical students today are called upon to integrate the basic and clinical sciences, in some cases from the first month of their curriculum. Students are often expected to complete self-directed study before meeting with other students in problem-based learning groups.

This book showcases the integration of basic and clinical science necessary to prepare for medical practice. It presents the alterations of structure and function that underlie disease, along with appropriate diagnostics and therapies. The book is not intended to be an exhaustive review of each organ system's pathologies, but rather a learning model for integrated mastery of USMLE Step 1 test systems.

The vignettes you will encounter represent the variety of core problems arising in a given system. They should be thought of as case exercises; they do not represent full clinical case presentations, but present enough information to allow you to generate a broad differential diagnosis.

Each chapter in the book covers an organ system. The chapters may be read in any order. To make the most of your study, we recommend the following:

- First, as a self-test, review the 10 patient vignettes and do your best to generate a differential diagnosis. As you consider your differential, keep in mind the list of diseases for that organ system.
- Then, work the chapters systematically. Begin with the checklist of diseases affecting an organ system. Next, move to the chapter vignettes, and then on to the disease discussions.
- Disease discussions begin with a pathogenesis section that names the correct diagnosis in the first sentence. Then the discussion moves on to disease-specific clinical presentation, diagnostic studies, morphologic findings, differential diagnosis, and treatment/outcomes along with integrated physiology and pharmacology correlations.
- Finally, test your knowledge of integration with the assessment questions at the end.

For **first year medical students**, this book will help with problem-based learning. For **second year medical students**, it will help to clarify the layers of finesse and integration needed to prepare for USMLE Step 1. For **third** and **fourth year students** it will serve as a reference when seeing patients during clinical rotations.

Student feedback has led us to create this resource, and it is only through continued feedback that this book will improve. We hope you will share your impressions by writing to us at medfeedback@kaplan.com.

Good luck in your studies.

Kaplan Medical

* As of this printing, all of the medical information contained herein is correct. However, clinical medicine changes daily. Note that on the exam you will not be tested on "brand new" practices.

CHAPTER 1

Hematopoietic and Lymphoreticular System

Checklist of Processes Within This System

Developmental Disorders

- ❏ Congenital thymic cyst
- ❏ Thymic hypoplasia
- ❏ Accessory spleen
- ❏ Fanconi anemia
- ❏ Diamond-Blackfan anemia

Infectious Diseases

- ❏ Splenic hydatidosis
- ❏ Infectious mononucleosis
- ❏ Cat-scratch disease
- ❏ Malaria
- ❏ CMV

Inflammatory Diseases

- ❏ Acquired multilocular thymic cyst
- ❏ Graft-versus-host disease

Autoimmune Diseases

- ❏ Autoimmune hemolytic anemia
- ❏ Immune thrombocytopenic purpura

Trauma

- ❏ Penetrating splenic injury
- ❏ Blunt splenic trauma

System-Specific Diseases

- ❏ Reactive changes in WBCs: leukocytosis and leukopenia
- ❏ Morphologic changes in RBCs
  - ○ Shape changes: elliptocytes, spherocytes, target cells, acanthocytes, echinocytes, schistocytes, bite cells, teardrop cells, sickle cells
  - ○ Red cell inclusions on microscopy: basophilic stipples, Howell-Jolly bodies, Pappenheimer bodies, ring sideroblasts, Heinz bodies
- ❏ Platelet disorders: thrombocytopenia
- ❏ Anemias: micro-, macro-, normocytic
- ❏ Extramedullary hematopoiesis
- ❏ Lymphadenopathy
- ❏ Splenomegaly

Neoplasia

- ❏ Lymphoid neoplasms: mature B cell neoplasms, peripheral T-cell and natural killer neoplasms, Hodgkin lymphoma, B and T lymphoblastic lymphoma/leukemia
- ❏ Myeloid neoplasms: acute myelogenous leukemia, myelodysplastic syndromes
- ❏ Myeloproliferative neoplasms: chronic myelogenous leukemia, polycythemia vera, essential thrombocythemia, myelofibrosis with myeloid metaplasia
- ❏ Multiple myeloma
- ❏ Localized extracutaneous mast cell neoplasms
- ❏ Splenic lymphangiomas and hemangiomas
- ❏ Thymomas
- ❏ Posttransplant lymphoproliferative disorder

Representative Diseases

What follows are clinical vignettes for 10 select diseases within this organ system. First, read the vignette and try to identify the condition. Then, move on to read integrated information on each disease.

Vignette 1

A full-term baby girl is born to a 23-year-old G1P0 mother who did not seek prenatal care. The newborn turns blue shortly after birth; she also has a cleft palate. Within a few hours of birth, she develops muscle spasms. Lab evaluation reveals a low CD3 count and low ionized calcium.

Diagnosis? _____

Vignette 2

A 54-year-old college professor notices that his face appears red and swollen. Physical examination is also notable for distended veins in his neck. Chest x-ray shows a well-circumscribed anterior mediastinal mass with no evidence of local invasion, lung mass, or lymphadenopathy.

Diagnosis? _____

Vignette 3

An 8-year-old boy presents to the pediatrician with yellow eyes, pale skin, and dark urine. His mother states that he began having upper respiratory symptoms 2 days ago. She also states that her brother has similar episodes when he gets a cold. CBC is notable for normocytic anemia, elevated bilirubin, and negative fluorescent spot test. Peripheral blood smear reveals Heinz bodies and bite cells.

Diagnosis? _____

Vignette 4

A father takes his 6-year-old son to the pediatrician because of several dark itchy lesions below the waistband of his shorts and under his socks. He is otherwise healthy. The father states the boy appears to scratch his legs more on hot days. Physical examination reveals many hyperpigmented patches that are most prominent around the waist and ankles.

Diagnosis? _____

Vignette 5

A 16-year-old boy presents with a high fever for several days. He also reveals that he has lost 10 pounds in the last 2 weeks. Physical examination reveals bilateral nontender lymphadenopathy. Imaging of the chest demonstrates a bulky anterior mediastinal mass.

Diagnosis? _____

Vignette 6

A 45-year-old woman presents to the ED with a spontaneous nosebleed. She reports 1 week of a fever that has not responded to acetaminophen. She denies cough, shortness of breath, abdominal pain, dysuria, and rash. Physical examination is notable for active bleeding from the nares bilaterally and numerous pinpoint red papules on her lower extremities. Lab evaluation reveals elevated white blood cell count, low hemoglobin/hematocrit, and low platelets.

Diagnosis? _____

Vignette 7

A 68-year-old man presents for an annual physical examination. He reports mild fatigue for several months but attributes this to "just getting older." Lab evaluation reveals microcytic anemia, undetectable ferritin, and thrombocytopenia.

Diagnosis? _____

Vignette 8

A 26-year-old woman presents to her primary care physician complaining of 1 year of heavy menses. On physical examination there are several red pinpoint macules on the buccal mucosa and there are ecchymoses on the extremities. Platelet count is 18,000/μL.

Diagnosis? _____

Vignette 9

A 50-year-old male smoker presents to the ED with a severe headache and dizziness. CBC is significant for hemoglobin 18.5 g/dL and urinalysis is positive for blood. Abdominal imaging reveals a renal mass.

Diagnosis? _____

Vignette 10

A 25-year-old man is playing with a new rescue cat he recently brought home. A few days later he develops a swollen red lesion on his left hand. Two weeks later he develops painful swelling in his left axilla and a fever.

Diagnosis? _____

Vignette 1

A full-term baby girl is born to a 23-year-old G1P0 mother who did not seek prenatal care. The newborn turns blue shortly after birth; she also has a cleft palate. Within a few hours of birth, she develops muscle spasms. Lab evaluation reveals a low CD3 count and low ionized calcium.

Pathogenesis. 22q11.2 deletion syndrome is also known as DiGeorge syndrome and velocardiofacial syndrome. It is caused by a microdeletion on chromosome 22 on the long ('q') arm at the 11.2 locus. This deletion leads to abnormal fetal development of 3rd and 4th pharyngeal pouches, which are involved with the development of the thymus and parathyroid glands. Most patients are heterozygotes; the disorder is usually sporadic but can be familial with autosomal dominant inheritance. It is one of the most common syndromes with multiple anomalies.

Clinical Presentation. The syndrome phenotype is highly variable. Children with the syndrome typically present with some combination of **cardiac malformation**, **thymic hypoplasia with immunodeficiency**, and **hypocalcemia** due to hypoparathyroidism. It is the most common syndrome associated with cleft palate. Cardiac malformations include tetralogy of Fallot, truncus arteriosus, and interrupted aortic arch, all of which cause cyanosis in the newborn period; ventricular septal defect (VSD) is the most common heart anomaly. Immunodeficiency can be mild or severe. Cognitive deficits are common, and there is an increased rate of psychiatric disorders including schizophrenia. Children with milder manifestations of DiGeorge may not be identified until later in childhood when they experience recurrent infections. Some cases may go undetected.

Diagnostic Studies.
- Molecular testing of amniotic fluid (prenatal) or blood (postnatal) for 22q11.2 deletion via FISH (fluorescence in situ hybridization) analysis
- Echocardiogram identifies specific cardiac anomalies
- Chest x-ray can identify **absence of thymic shadow**
- **Low CD3(+) T-cell count** confirms immunodeficiency
- Low ionized/free calcium with inappropriately low parathyroid hormone
- Pulse oximetry identifies hypoxemia even in the absence of frank cyanosis

Morphologic Features.
- Gross examination: heart malformations (tetralogy of Fallot, truncus arteriosus, or interrupted aortic arch), cleft palate
- Microscopic: depletion of T-cell zones of lymphoid organs

Differential Diagnosis. Any of the syndromic features can be present in isolation. Patients with prenatal exposure to ethanol or retinoids can have a DiGeorge-like phenotype, but will lack the 22q11.2 deletion. HIV can also cause isolated T-cell deficiency, but congenital HIV would not be associated with heart malformations or hypocalcemia.

Treatment and Outcomes.
- Stem cell or thymic transplant for severely immunosuppressed children
- Surgical repair of cleft palate and cyanotic heart malformations; facial reconstructive surgery
- Calcium replacement therapy administered with activated vitamin D
- Prognosis and life expectancy depend on severity of cardiac malformation and immunosuppression

Physiology Correlation. In response to low ionized calcium in the blood, the parathyroid glands secrete parathyroid hormone (PTH). PTH increases serum calcium by acting in the kidneys and the bones. In the kidneys, PTH binds to calcium channels in the distal tubule, causing them to open and allow more calcium reabsorption. In the bone, PTH binds to osteoblasts, causing them to activate osteoclasts. Increased osteoclastic activity releases calcium and phosphate from the bone, termed *resorption.*

Pharmacology Correlation. Vitamin D is ingested in one of 2 inactive forms: D2 (ergocalciferol) or D3 (cholecalciferol). Both forms are converted in the liver to 25-OH vitamin D, which is subsequently converted to the final active form 1, 25-dihydroxyvitamin D (calcitriol) in the kidneys by α1-hydroxylase. Calcitriol increases blood calcium levels by increasing calcium absorption from the GI tract and the distal tubules of the kidney. Calcitriol works in conjunction with PTH by increasing production of calbindin, a calcium binding protein, within the tubular epithelial cells to facilitate reabsorption.

Vignette 2

A 54-year-old college professor notices that his face appears red and swollen. Physical examination is also notable for distended veins in his neck. Chest x-ray shows a well-circumscribed anterior mediastinal mass with no evidence of local invasion, lung mass, or lymphadenopathy.

Pathogenesis. A **thymoma** is a benign **epithelial neoplasm** arising in the thymus. It represents about half of all tumors arising in the anterior mediastinum. Because thymomas release immature T-cells into the circulation, this neoplasm is associated with autoimmune disorders. About a third of patients with thymoma also have **myasthenia gravis** (MG).

Clinical Presentation. Thymoma typically presents in decades 4 or 5 of life. Patients may experience signs and symptoms of superior vena cava syndrome, including facial plethora and swelling, distension of neck veins, and upper extremity swelling. Other symptoms of a mediastinal mass may include chest pain or dyspnea. Patients may also present with symptoms of MG, including facial or limb weakness; thymic abnormalities are present in 75% of all AChR antibody–positive MG patients. A minority of patients with thymoma are asymptomatic and the tumor is an incidental finding during imaging studies.

Diagnostic Studies.
- Chest CT or MRI can confirm the presence of a mediastinal mass and determine whether resection is possible.
- If MG is suspected, the edrophonium test is only administered if antibody and electrodiagnostic test results are negative.
- **AchR antibodies** are positive in most patients with a thymoma and MG.

Morphologic Features.
- Gross examination: firm gray-white mass ranging in size up to 20 cm. Cytologically benign thymomas may be noninvasive or invasive.
- Microscopic: The tumors are morphologically heterogeneous and consist of a mixture of thymic epithelial cells without atypia and lymphocytes. Perivascular clearing (a hypocellular area around venules) is a predominant feature of one of the subtypes. Thymic carcinomas (5% of thymomas) are usually squamous cell carcinomas.

Differential Diagnosis. In adults, **most mediastinal tumors are anterior and malignant.** Thymic carcinoma will show signs of invasion on chest imaging. If resected, it will be infiltrative rather than circumscribed. Lymphomas can involve the mediastinum but usually demonstrate extramediastinal involvement. Germ cell tumors of the mediastinum can be associated with elevated hCG and/ or AFP.

Treatment and Outcomes.

- **Thymectomy** if possible
- Chemotherapy and/or radiation if mass is unresectable
- Most patients with a resectable mass have an excellent prognosis and rarely have recurrences

Physiology Correlation. Superior vena cava (SVC) syndrome develops when the SVC is compressed by a mediastinal or lung mass. When the SVC is compressed, blood flow from all veins that empty into the SVC (including brachiocephalic, jugular, and subclavian veins) is obstructed. Thus the anatomical sites drained by these veins become congested with blood, leading to swelling, redness, and prominent veins in the head, upper extremity, and upper chest.

Pharmacology Correlation. Acetylcholinesterase (AChE) inhibitors such as pyridostigmine or neostigmine are cholinergic agonists commonly used to treat MG. AChE normally breaks down acetylcholine at the neuromuscular junction. When AChE is blocked, the concentration of acetylcholine increases in the neuromuscular junction, temporarily overcoming the inhibitory action of the anti-AChR antibodies.

Vignette 3

An 8-year-old boy presents to the pediatrician with yellow eyes, pale skin, and dark urine. His mother states that he began having upper respiratory symptoms 2 days ago. She also states that her brother has similar episodes when he gets a cold. CBC is notable for normocytic anemia, elevated bilirubin, and negative fluorescent spot test. Peripheral blood smear reveals Heinz bodies and bite cells.

Pathogenesis. Glucose-6 phosphate dehydrogenase deficiency (or G6PD deficiency) is an X-linked recessive disorder of RBC metabolism. There are hundreds of variants. At the subcellular level there is an inability to produce enough NADPH to reduce glutathione. RBCs which lack G6PD are sensitive to oxidative stress, resulting in periodic hemolysis. The disease is common in males of African and Mediterranean origin.

Clinical Presentation. Patients present with anemia, hyperbilirubinemia, methemoglobinemia, and hemoglobinuria. Triggers for hemolysis include infection, ingestion of fava beans, and exposure to oxidizing medications. Patients usually do not have chronic, baseline hemolysis.

Diagnostic Studies.
- CBC shows **normocytic anemia** (MCV 80–100)
- Elevated total and direct bilirubin (extravascular hemolysis)
- Fluorescent spot test: negative due to NADPH deficiency
- Quantitative biochemical G6PD assay. Measurement during acute hemolysis may cause false negative results.

Morphologic Features.
- Peripheral blood smear: **Heinz bodies** (oxidized hemoglobin), **bite cells**

Differential Diagnosis. Sickle cell disease (SCD) also causes hemolysis in individuals of African and Mediterranean origin. Patients with SCD usually have chronic baseline hemolysis, unlike G6PD-deficient patients. Their peripheral blood smear shows sickled cells, not bite cells. Hemoglobin electrophoresis reveals abnormal hemoglobin S.

Treatment and Outcomes.
- Treatment of underlying infection if applicable
- Avoidance of medications that trigger hemolysis
- Discontinuation of inciting medications
- Hydration of patient during hemolytic episode
- Normal life expectancy

Physiology Correlation. G6PD synthesizes NADPH and reduced glutathione (GSH) in the hexose monophosphate shunt; they provide protection against antioxidants. In the absence of G6PD, RBCs are sensitive to oxidative stress. As hemoglobin oxidizes, it precipitates into Heinz bodies that are cleared by the spleen, leaving 'bite' cells.

Pharmacology Correlation. Primaquine, a quinoline derivative, is an antimalarial drug that can be used for primary prophylaxis or treatment. It attacks not only the intraerythrocytic form of the parasite but also intrahepatic parasites (hypnozoites) and gametocytes. Primaquine, along with other oxidizing medications such as methylene blue, sulfa drugs, and nitrofurantoin, should be avoided in patients with G6PD deficiency.

Vignette 4

A father takes his 6-year-old son to the pediatrician because of several dark itchy lesions below the waistband of his shorts and under his socks. He is otherwise healthy. The father states the boy appears to scratch his legs more on hot days. Physical examination reveals many hyperpigmented patches that are most prominent around the waist and ankles.

Pathogenesis. Cutaneous mastocytosis is a condition characterized by increased numbers of mast cells in the skin due to a mutation in the *KIT* gene. The excess mast cells degranulate, releasing histamine, which causes intense pruritus. The most common form of the condition is **urticaria pigmentosa**.

Clinical Presentation. Cutaneous mastocytosis is usually seen in children who present with severe pruritus after exposure to triggers such as local irritation or heat, like the child in vignette 4 who is most affected at the site of tight-fitting clothing. Bullae or pigmented macules/patches may develop. **Darier's sign** is typically positive; upon stroking an area of the skin, erythema, urticaria, and pruritus develop at the site within minutes.

Diagnostic Studies.
- **Elevated serum tryptase**
- CBC is normal
- Molecular testing reveals **mutation of the *KIT* gene**

Morphologic Features.
- Microscopic: numerous mast cells (mononuclear cells with heavy basophilic granulation) in the epidermis which **stain positive for tryptase**

Differential Diagnosis. Children with localized pruritus are much more likely to have atopic dermatitis or irritant dermatitis than cutaneous mastocytosis. These disorders are more likely to cause an eczematous-type rash with thick, scaling skin rather than discrete lesions. Diffuse urticaria or pruritus are more likely to reflect an allergic condition than mastocytosis. Systemic mastocytosis can also involve the skin, but is defined by involvement of several organ systems; laboratory abnormalities often include anemia and thrombocytopenia.

Treatment and Outcomes.

- Anaphylaxis is a rare occurrence (treatment with epinephrine injection).
- Antihistamines, specifically H1 blockers (diphenhydramine, cetirizine, loratadine), can be useful for treating pruritus.
- Avoidance of triggers is an important part of recovery.
- Resolution over time is expected with few to no long-term sequelae.

Physiology Correlation. Type I, or immediate type, **hypersensitivity reactions** require at least 2 exposures to the allergic trigger: initial exposure that sensitizes the individual, and subsequent exposure that triggers the hypersensitivity reaction. After the initial exposure, type 2 helper T cells (Th2 cells) stimulate B cells to synthesize IgE that binds to mast cell Fc receptors. Upon re-exposure, the allergic trigger causes the IgE chains to crosslink, which stimulates the bound mast cells to degranulate. The release of histamine, heparin, and other mast cell granule contents results in local allergic-type symptoms including urticaria, rhinitis, and bronchoconstriction within a few hours of the exposure.

Pharmacology Correlation. Antihistamines, specifically **H1 antagonists**, block the action of histamine that is released from mast cells by competitively inhibiting at the histamine receptor sites. They can be useful in treating urticaria and pruritus associated with cutaneous mastocytosis. H1 antagonists for urticaria include diphenhydramine, cetirizine, loratadine, and fexofenadine. The most common side effect is sedation, particularly with diphenhydramine.

Vignette 5

A 16-year-old boy presents with a high fever for several days. He also reveals that he has lost 10 pounds in the last 2 weeks. Physical examination reveals bilateral nontender lymphadenopathy. Imaging of the chest demonstrates a bulky anterior mediastinal mass.

Pathogenesis. **T-cell lymphoblastic lymphoma** is a clonal neoplasm arising from T-lymphoid precursor cells. Many cases are associated with gain-of-function **mutations in the *NOTCH1* gene**. The NOTCH1 protein is normally a receptor involved with proliferation and maturation of T-lymphocytes in the thymus. Mutant NOTCH1 promotes overgrowth of T-cells by upregulating transcription factors such as c-myc, which increases the risk of development of a malignant clone.

Clinical Presentation. T-cell lymphoblastic lymphoma most often affects adolescents or young adults; it is slightly more common in males. Patients often present with typical "B symptoms" including fever, night sweats, and weight loss. Approximately 50% present with a mediastinal mass.

Diagnostic Studies.
- Chest CT or MRI demonstrates mediastinal mass and extensive lymphadenopathy
- Biopsy of lymph node or mediastinal mass
- Lumbar puncture is performed to rule out CNS involvement

Morphologic Features.
- Microscopy, lymph node/mediastinal mass: sheets of mitotically-active blasts with high nuclear-to-cytoplasmic ratio that obliterate normal lymphoid architecture
- Microscopy, bone marrow: **<25% blasts** that are **positive for TdT, CD7, CD2, and CD3, and negative for MPO** (by immunohistochemical stain or flow cytometry)

Differential Diagnosis. If a patient's bone marrow demonstrates >25% blasts, lymphoblastic leukemia rather than lymphoma is diagnosed. Many mediastinal masses start with a *t*:
- Terrible lymphoma (i.e., lymphoblastic lymphoma)
- Thymoma
- Teratoma
- Thyromegaly (goiter)

Thymomas are usually well-circumscribed and not associated with widespread lymphadenopathy. Teratomas may be heterogeneous on imaging with bony and fatty components. Thyroid enlargement is usually evident on physical examination and may occasionally extend inferiorly into the mediastinum.

Treatment and Outcomes.

- Treatment includes chemotherapy, radiation, and allogeneic stem cell transplantation
- Outcome depends on patient's age: children with ALL have a 5-year survival rate of 85% but prognosis is worse with advancing age

Physiology Correlation. T cell activation is part of the adaptive immune response, whose endpoints are production of antibodies and direct killing of microbes. CD4+ T cells help B cells make antibodies; CD8+ T cells kill cells that express foreign antigen. Class II MHC molecules allow CD4+ T cells to recognize foreign peptides. Class I MHC molecules interact with CD8+ T cells. You can remember these associations because $2 \times 4 = 8$ and $1 \times 8 = 8$.

Pharmacology Correlation. Cyclophosphamide is a chemotherapeutic agent often used to treat lymphoblastic lymphoma, and many other hematologic malignancies. It is an alkylating agent that targets guanine nucleotides, rendering DNA unable to replicate. In addition to bone marrow suppression, which is a common side effect of many chemotherapeutics, **cyclophosphamide causes hemorrhagic cystitis** in a dose-dependent fashion. Mesna, which binds the toxic metabolite responsible for hemorrhagic cystitis, is given prophylactically to patients treated with cyclophosphamide.

Vignette 6

A 45-year-old woman presents to the ED with a spontaneous nosebleed. She reports 1 week of a fever that has not responded to acetaminophen. She denies cough, shortness of breath, abdominal pain, dysuria, and rash. Physical examination is notable for active bleeding from the nares bilaterally and numerous pinpoint red papules on her lower extremities. Lab evaluation reveals elevated white blood cell count, low hemoglobin/hematocrit, and low platelets.

Pathogenesis. Acute myeloid leukemia (AML), also known as acute myelogenous leukemia, is a clonal neoplasm arising from myeloid precursor cells. There are a plethora of subtypes distinguished by molecular abnormalities and immunophenotype. One distinctive subtype is acute promyelocytic leukemia, or APL, which arises from promyelocytes.

Clinical Presentation. AML is typically a malignancy of middle-aged adults. Presentation includes vague systemic symptoms including fatigue, fever, and weight loss, plus elevated white blood cell count with anemia and thrombocytopenia. Patients with APL often present with disseminated intravascular coagulation (DIC), which causes bleeding as seen in the vignette and paradoxical concomitant clotting.

Diagnostic Studies.
- CBC demonstrates **leukocytosis with predominately blasts** (large WBCs with nucleomegaly and prominent nucleoli), anemia, and thrombocytopenia.
- Cytogenetics identifies classic translocations in many subtypes; **t(15;17)** *PML-RARA* is seen in APL.

Morphologic Features.
- Peripheral blood smear: blasts with cytoplasmic **Auer rods** (red-violet stick-like inclusions)
- Microscopy, bone marrow, AML: >20% blasts that are positive for MPO, CD34
- Microscopy, bone marrow, APL: >20% blasts that are positive for CD13, CD33

Differential Diagnosis. On peripheral blood smear, it is impossible to distinguish myeloblasts from lymphoblasts unless Auer rods are seen (they are never seen in lymphoblasts). Acute lymphoblastic leukemia (ALL) more commonly affects children but can rarely affect adults. Determining the immunophenotype of the blasts, either by flow cytometry or staining of the bone marrow biopsy, clarifies the lineage of the blasts.

Treatment and Outcomes.
- DIC is a medical emergency. Untreated APL with DIC is usually rapidly fatal due to hemorrhage.
- The 5-year survival for adults is about 25%, but prognosis varies with age and molecular features.
- Molecular/cytogenetic abnormalities
  - t(15;17) *PML-RARA* in APL: better prognosis, treated with all-trans retinoic acid (ATRA; a vitamin A analog)
  - *FLT3* mutation: worse prognosis

Physiology Correlation. Hemostasis is the complex process by which a mature thrombus forms through the interaction of platelets and coagulation factors. Upon vascular endothelial damage, GPIb on the surface of platelets binds to von Willebrand factor bound to the endothelial wall. Platelet activation is stimulated by ADP, epinephrine, and thrombin. Fibrinogen binding to GPIIb-IIIa aggregates platelets together by crosslinking multiple platelets. Fibrinogen is the end product of the coagulation cascade, in which coagulation factors sequentially activate each other.

Pharmacology Correlation. All-trans retinoic acid (ATRA) is used to treat APL. ATRA targets the product of the fusion protein created by the translocation t(15;17) which involves retinoic acid receptor alpha (RARA). Upon binding to RARA, ATRA causes maturation and differentiation of the malignant promyelocytes into mature myelocytes. Side effects often occur together in "differentiation syndrome" (seen in 25% of patients), and include fever, acute respiratory distress, and pleural and/or pericardial effusion.

Vignette 7

A 68-year-old man presents for an annual physical examination. He reports mild fatigue for several months but attributes this to "just getting older." Lab evaluation reveals microcytic anemia, undetectable ferritin, and thrombocytopenia.

Pathogenesis. **Myelodysplastic syndrome** (MDS) is a clonal stem cell disorder. For primary MDS, mean age is >50, while for secondary MDS mean age is young adulthood in patients postchemotherapy/radiation or with a heritable disorder of DNA repair such as Fanconi anemia.

Clinical Presentation. MDS is usually a disease of older adults with a slight male predominance. Patients are often asymptomatic and diagnosed when routine laboratory studies demonstrate cytopenias. Symptoms of anemia such as fatigue, shortness of breath, dizziness on standing, or chest pain may also be present at diagnosis.

Diagnostic Studies.
- CBC shows anemia in a majority of patients with MDS. Leukopenia and/or thrombocytopenia may be present.
- Bone marrow biopsy is required for diagnosis.

Morphologic Features.
- Microscopic, peripheral blood: nucleated red blood cells with basophilic stippling (ribosomal inclusions) or Howell-Jolly bodies (DNA inclusions)
- Microscopic, bone marrow: hypercellular with **<20% blasts,** fibrosis, and dysplasia in at least one cell line: **Pelger-Huet cells** (WBCs with bilobed nuclei shaped like aviator sunglasses), **ringed sideroblasts** (RBC precursors with iron granules), and **"pawn ball" megakaryocytes** (trilobed nuclei).

Differential Diagnosis. Myeloproliferative neoplasms (MPN) are clonal disorders of one bone marrow cell line: essential thrombocytosis (ET), polycythemia vera (PV), and chronic myeloid leukemia (CML). These disorders have classic molecular abnormalities: CML with t(9;22), the Philadelphia chromosome; PV with *JAK2* mutation.

Treatment and Outcomes.

- Treatment varies depending on severity of clinical manifestations. Patients may be treated conservatively with blood transfusions to manage cytopenias or more aggressively with a variety of chemotherapeutic agents.
- Patients with a high risk of progression may be treated with stem cell transplant.
- Risk of progression to acute myeloid leukemia increases as blast count approaches 20%. Progression to AML is a poor prognostic sign.
- Risk of death is higher in patients with blast count >10%, severe cytopenia(s), complex karyotype, and older age.

Physiology Correlation. Ferrous iron (Fe^{2+}; "2 of us") is absorbed in the duodenum. Absorption is enhanced by coingestion of vitamin C and inhibited by coingestion of calcium, another divalent cation. After entering the bloodstream via ferroportin on the luminal surface of duodenal enterocytes, iron binds to transferrin. Transferrin can move iron to the bone marrow for storage as ferritin. As transferrin saturation increases, hepatocytes synthesize more hepcidin, a protein that inhibits iron absorption to prevent iron overload.

Pharmacology Correlation. Chronically anemic patients who receive many red blood cell transfusions are at risk for iron overload. Other than menstruation, there is no physiologic method of excreting iron; thus iron chelation therapy can be implemented in patients who demonstrate evidence of iron overload. Deferoxamine and other chelators bind to iron, and the complex is then excreted in urine and feces.

Vignette 8

A 26-year-old woman presents to her primary care physician complaining of 1 year of heavy menses. On physical examination there are several red pinpoint macules on the buccal mucosa and there are ecchymoses on the extremities. Platelet count is 18,000/μL.

Pathogenesis. Chronic immune thrombocytopenic purpura (ITP), previously known as idiopathic thrombocytopenia purpura, is a type II hypersensitivity reaction in which autoantibodies target platelet antigens (usually GPIIb-III or GPIb). These antibody-coated platelets are then cleared by the spleen, causing thrombocytopenia.

Clinical Presentation. ITP can be acute or chronic. Acute ITP is seen in children following a viral infection. Chronic ITP is more common in women of child-bearing age (like most autoimmune diseases) and presents with menorrhagia, epistaxis, bruising, and petechiae. Patients often have platelet counts below 20,000, as in the vignette. By definition, chronic ITP must have a duration of at least 3 months.

Diagnostic Studies.
- CBC shows **isolated thrombocytopenia.**
- PT/INR, PTT, fibrinogen are all normal.
- Bone marrow biopsy is usually not performed.

Morphologic Features.
- Microscopy, bone marrow: increased number of megakaryocytes

Differential Diagnosis. Thrombotic thrombocytopenic purpura (TTP) can be associated with acute onset thrombocytopenia, but typically also includes some combination of hemolytic anemia, neurological symptoms, fever, and acute kidney injury. Aplastic anemia due to infection or medication causes thrombocytopenia, but RBCs and WBCs are usually reduced as well.

Treatment and Outcomes.
- Acute ITP is usually self-limited and unlikely to recur.
- Corticosteroids and intravenous immunoglobulin (IVIG) are mainstays of therapy for chronic ITP; splenectomy is second-line.
- Platelet transfusion is reserved for patients with ITP who are actively bleeding.

Physiology Correlation. In type II hypersensitivity reactions, autoanti-bodies directed at specific cell types are synthesized. As the targeted cells become coated with antibodies, they are either cleared by the spleen if they are bloodborne or cause local damage if located within tissue. The effects are organ- or cell-specific rather than systemic.

Pharmacology Correlation. IVIG is used to treat many autoimmune disor-ders. This medication is made by pooling purified immunoglobulins from thousands of healthy blood donors. While the exact mechanism is unknown, it is theorized that adding an excess of immunoglobulins creates a negative feedback loop, preventing the patient's immune system from synthesizing more pathological autoantibodies.

Vignette 9

A 50-year-old male smoker presents to the ED with a severe headache and dizziness. CBC is significant for hemoglobin 18.5 g/dL and urinalysis is positive for blood. Abdominal imaging reveals a renal mass.

Pathogenesis. Paraneoplastic hematologic syndrome occurs in about 3% of patients with renal cell carcinoma. In cases with **erythrocytosis**, tumor secretion of EPO causes the bone marrow to produce more RBCs, and the hematocrit increases.

Clinical Presentation. Patients with polycythemia of any cause often present with dizziness, headache, or stroke. Renal cell carcinoma can also present with hematuria, flank pain, and a palpable abdominal mass. The paraneoplastic syndrome may be the initial presentation of the underlying malignancy.

Diagnostic Studies.
- CBC shows **elevation of hematocrit**
- Workup for patients with erythrocytosis and a cancer known to cause erythrocytosis (e.g., renal cell carcinoma or hepatocellular carcinoma), includes measurement of red blood cell mass and serum erythropoietin level

Morphologic Features.
- Kidney tumor: a renal cell carcinoma typically arises in one pole of the kidney and has a yellow cut surface and tumor cells with a granular or clear cytoplasm due to the lipid content.
- Microscopic features of bone marrow in paraneoplastic erythrocytosis
  - Hyperplasia of erythroid precursors with normal-appearing white blood cell precursors and megakaryocytes
  - No dysplasia or fibrosis (ruling out polycythemia vera)

Differential Diagnosis. Polycythemia vera (PV), a myeloproliferative disorder affecting the erythroid lineage, is associated with *JAK2* mutation, which is absent in paraneoplastic polycythemia. Hereditary hemochromatosis also causes elevated hemoglobin/hematocrit and is often associated with hyperpigmented skin and new-onset diabetes ("bronze diabetes"). Hematuria in a smoker is concerning for bladder cancer, but this malignancy is not associated with polycythemia.

Treatment and Outcomes.

- Tumor resection usually resolves the paraneoplastic syndrome.
- If treatment of the underlying malignancy is not effective, therapeutic phlebotomy may control symptoms.

Physiology Correlation. Under hypoxemic conditions, EPO is secreted in the kidney. In response to EPO secretion, the bone marrow responds by increasing erythropoiesis (RBC synthesis) to increase the oxygen-carrying capacity of the blood. The increased RBC content of the blood then signals the kidney to reduce EPO synthesis in a negative feedback loop.

Pharmacology Correlation. EPO can be used to treat patients who are anemic because of chemotherapy or chronic kidney disease. These patients are often chronically anemic, and EPO can help reduce the need for blood transfusions. Concurrent supplemental iron may be required to ensure adequate erythropoiesis.

Vignette 10

A 25-year-old man is playing with a new rescue cat he recently brought home. A few days later he develops a swollen red lesion on his left hand. Two weeks later he develops painful swelling in his left axilla and a fever.

Pathogenesis. ***Bartonella henselae*** is a zoonotic pathogen that causes both **cat scratch disease/fever** and **bacillary angiomatosis** in AIDS patients. Many cats are carriers of *B. henselae* and can become infected via flea bite. Rarely, and for unknown reasons, cat scratch disease progresses to neurological or disseminated infection in immunocompetent hosts.

Clinical Presentation. Patients have a history of a cat scratch approximately 1 week prior to developing an erythematous papule at that site. Tender lymphadenopathy develops about 2 weeks after the scratch in the nodes draining the area of initial inoculation. Despite the name "cat scratch fever," not all patients are febrile.

Diagnostic Studies.
- Clinical presentation and history are typically sufficient for diagnosis.
- Serologic testing for anti-*Bartonella* IgM antibodies is diagnostic.
- Blood culture on chocolate agar to enhance growth of this fastidious organism. Gram stain reveals gram-negative rods.
- Lymph node biopsy may be useful to rule out other disorders if the diagnosis is unclear.

Morphologic Features.
- Microscopy, lymph node: necrotizing granulomas
- Organisms are Warthin-Starry-positive and AFB-negative

Differential Diagnosis. Hodgkin lymphoma could also cause regional lymphadenopathy and fever in a young adult, but the involved node(s) will not be tender. If necrotizing granulomas are seen on histology, tuberculosis is ruled out with an AFB (acid-fast bacillus) stain. Other gram-negative rods associated with bites include *Capnocytophaga canimorsus* (dog bites; "cani-" = dog; "-morsus" = mouth) and *Eikenella corrodens* (human bites; agar plate appears pitted with bleach-like odor). Both of these pathogens cause cellulitis at the site of the bite. The classic history of specific exposures helps distinguish between these pathogens.

Treatment and Outcomes.

- Azithromycin or doxycycline (typically allows full recovery with no long-term sequelae)
- Spontaneous resolution without treatment in some cases

Physiology Correlation. Granulomas (or granulomatous inflammation) are one type of inflammatory response. Pathogens including tuberculosis, fungi, or *Bartonella* species typically elicit a granulomatous response, as do foreign bodies such as splinters or retained sutures. Macrophages surround the offending agent in an attempt to protect the rest of the body from becoming exposed.

Pharmacology Correlation. Doxycycline can be used to treat several zoonotic or vector-borne illnesses. This tetracycline antibiotic is bacteriostatic, inhibiting protein synthesis. It is often given prophylactically after a human or animal bite. It can be used to treat many infections transmitted by insects including Lyme disease (*Borrelia burgdorferi*; tick bite), Rocky Mountain spotted fever (*Rickettsia*; tick bite), tularemia (*Francisella tularensis*; deer fly bite), and plague (*Yersinia pestis*; flea bite).

Test What You Have Learned

1. Ultrasound-guided biopsy of a 4 cm mediastinal mass is obtained from a 13-year-old boy who was evaluated for shortness of breath, fever, and night sweats. The biopsy demonstrates that a large lymph node has been overrun with sheets of mitotically active blasts with high nuclear-to-cytoplasmic ratio. These cells would most likely be associated with an abnormality involving which of the following?

    A. 22q11.2

    B. JAK2

    C. KIT

    D. NOTCH1

    E. RARA

    F. t(9;22)

2. Routine blood evaluation of a 54-year-old woman demonstrates microcytic anemia and thrombocytopenia. On questioning, the patient has been experiencing a low level of fatigue, but she is without other complaints. Review of the peripheral smear is notable for the presence of nucleated red blood cells with basophilic stippling and Howell-Jolly bodies. If this patient's disease progresses over time to the point of requiring multiple transfusions, which of the following medications would be most likely to be used to chelate iron to reduce a possible iron overload?

    A. ATRA

    B. Deferoxamine

    C. Doxycycline

    D. EPO

    E. IV immunoglobulin

    F. Mesna

3. An 8-year-old girl visits a dermatologist for evaluation of a tendency to develop skin manifestations after playing outdoors in the summer. The child complains of being very itchy when she gets too warm. Examination demonstrates both bullae and pigmented macules around the waist and lower legs. Punch biopsy of one of these lesions would most likely demonstrate which of the following?

   A. Auer rods

   B. Heinz bodies

   C. Increased megakaryocytes

   D. Low CD3 count

   E. Positive staining for tryptase

   F. Ringed sideroblasts

4. A full-term newborn boy has a cleft palate. Shortly after birth, the baby develops muscle spasms. The neonate's initial blood work is notable for a low ionized calcium. Which of the following would be most likely to be also found on further evaluation?

   A. Axillary mass in lymph node

   B. Anterior mediastinal mass

   C. Autoantibodies to platelet antigens

   D. Blast cells in bone marrow

   E. Darier's sign

   F. No thymic shadow

5. Following a minor automobile accident, a 32-year-old woman is taken to the local ED. While there she is noted to have more large bruises than would be expected by the seriousness of the accident. She also describes several years of heavy menstrual periods. CBC studies show an isolated thrombocytopenia. PT/INR, PTT, and fibrinogen are all normal. Given this presentation, the patient is most likely to also have which of the following?

   A. Anti-Barton antibodies

   B. Anti- GPIIb-III antibodies

   C. Diffuse urticaria

   D. Paraneoplastic myasthenia gravis

   E. Severe combined immunodeficiency

   F. T cell deficiency

Answers: 1. (D), 2. (B), 3. (E), 4. (F), 5. (B).

CHAPTER 2
Nervous System and Special Senses

Developmental Disorders

❏ Fetal alcohol syndrome
❏ Spina bifida
❏ Anencephaly
❏ Encephalocele
❏ Periventricular leukomalacia
❏ Coloboma

Infectious Diseases

❏ Meningitis
❏ Encephalitis
❏ Prion disease
❏ Conjunctivitis
❏ Brain abscess

Autoimmune Diseases

❏ Multiple sclerosis
❏ Sydenham's chorea

Trauma

❏ Diffuse axonal injury
❏ Subarachnoid hemorrhage
❏ Epidural/subdural hemorrhage
❏ Complete/incomplete spinal cord injury
❏ Complex regional pain syndrome

System-Specific Processes

❏ Cerebrovascular disease
  ° Hypertensive
  ° Vascular malformations
❏ Fluid increases
  ° Cerebral edema
  ° Hydrocephalus

❏ Increased intracranial pressure and herniation
❏ Demyelinating disease: MS; acute disseminated encephalomyelitis
❏ Leukodystrophies
❏ Degenerative disease: Alzheimer; Pick; Parkinson; Huntington; Friedreich ataxia; ALS
❏ Intracranial hemorrhage
❏ Lysosomal storage disease: Niemann-Pick; Gaucher; Tay-Sachs; Hurler and Hunter syndromes
❏ Dysautonomia: orthostatic hypotension; POTS; syncope
❏ Reactions to Toxins: ethanol; metals; chemicals; carbon monoxide; environmental toxins
❏ Ménière's disease
❏ Glaucoma

Neoplasia

❏ Choroidal melanoma
❏ Astrocytoma, anaplastic astrocytoma, glioblastoma
❏ Oligodendroglioma
❏ Ependymomas
❏ Medulloblastoma
❏ Meningioma
❏ Schwannoma
❏ Neurofibrosarcoma

Representative Diseases

What follows are clinical vignettes for 10 select diseases within this organ system. First, read the vignette and try to identify the condition. Then, move on to read integrated information on each disease.

Vignette 1

A 10-year-old boy with a known diagnosis of attention-deficit hyperactivity disorder experiences new onset of tonic-clonic seizures. EEG reveals diffuse spike-and-wave complexes. MRI reveals brain atrophy and hypoplasia of the corpus callosum.

Diagnosis? _____

Vignette 2

A 35-year-old man is involved in a ski accident in Colorado in the month of December. He returns home to Texas shortly thereafter, but begins to suffer from headaches. One day in January he tells his wife he cannot see, and she calls EMS.

Diagnosis? _____

Vignette 3

A 43-year-old public health professor develops limb weakness and an ascending paralysis. She recently traveled to Haiti.

Diagnosis? _____

Vignette 4

A 7-year-old boy presents to the doctor due to new onset of seizures. The mother reports that he has been falling down and "walking clumsily" for 6 months. He has also been performing poorly in school. The family history is uncertain due to adoption.

Diagnosis? _____

Vignette 5

A 35-year-old man asks his fiancé to drive him to urgent care after 3 hours of dizziness, vomiting, and imbalance. Before he can see the doctor, he collapses in the parking lot.

Diagnosis? _____

Vignette 6

A man in his 40s moves back to the United States from London and begins to feel depressed. He seeks help from a psychiatrist but withholds symptoms of memory loss. Following the onset of ataxia, he is referred to a neurologist. MRI reveals pulvinar sign. He dies 14 months later. Autopsy shows florid plaques.

Diagnosis? _____

Vignette 7

A 55-year-old man who was previously treated with radiation for head and neck cancer develops a new onset of headaches. He subsequently undergoes neuroimaging, and 2 parasagittal dural-based lesions are identified.

Diagnosis? _____

Vignette 8

A 28-year-old man is in his second month of treatment for tuberculosis when he begins to experience cognitive difficulty at work. A few weeks later, he has a generalized seizure at his office. A coworker drives him to the hospital, where a brain CT shows several ring-enhancing lesions.

Diagnosis? _____

Vignette 9

A 40-year-old man begins to have attacks of dizziness that cause him to lie down in bed. The attacks are accompanied by nausea and vomiting. When he seeks help from his doctor, he reports that he has also been experiencing episodic fluctuations in hearing, as well as ringing in the right ear.

Diagnosis? _____

Vignette 10

After a brief viral illness, a 16-year-old girl begins to suffer from episodes of tachycardia, lightheadedness, and brain fog. The symptoms persist for months, and her pediatrician refers her to a cardiologist. A tilt table test is performed.

Diagnosis? _____

Vignette 1

A 10-year-old boy with a known diagnosis of attention-deficit hyperactivity disorder experiences new onset of tonic-clonic seizures. EEG reveals diffuse spike-and-wave complexes. MRI reveals brain atrophy and hypoplasia of the corpus callosum.

Pathogenesis. Fetal alcohol syndrome (FAS) is the most severe end of the fetal alcohol spectrum that affects 1 in 100 children born in the United States. Alcohol is a teratogen, and maternal consumption of alcohol will have varying effects on the fetus depending on the timing, amount of use, and maternal sociobehavioral/genetic factors. The offspring of sexually active women who consume alcohol and do not use birth control are at risk for alcohol-related birth defects, alcohol-related neurodevelopmental disorders, partial FAS, and FAS. Alcohol causes **craniofacial dysmorphology** by interfering with neural crest migration. Ethanol diminishes the cytokine release that is necessary for neural growth. Alcohol disrupts neural stem cell function by altering the Wnt signaling pathway.

- Binge drinking causes a dose-related risk to the fetus.
- Comorbid conditions such as malnutrition can worsen the effects.
- Women who smoke and women from lower socioeconomic backgrounds are at higher risk.
- The risk of FAS is decreased in women with an efficient alcohol dehydrogenase enzyme.

Clinical Presentation. The effects of maternal alcohol consumption can be seen in craniofacial dysmorphology, central nervous system abnormalities, internal organ damage, development deficits, and growth retardation. Severe malformations (e.g., Dandy-Walker) also occur. Facial characteristics include small chin, cleft lip/palate, low nasal bridge, hypoplastic maxillae, ptosis, hypertelorism, prominent epicanthic fold, short nose/anteverted nostrils, short palpebral fissure, thin vermillion border of upper lip, and smooth philtrum (with the last three bearing diagnostic importance). Epilepsy is more prevalent in children with FAS. For the patient in the vignette, the workup for epilepsy led to further investigation, resulting in a diagnosis of FAS. Many cases are not diagnosed until school age due to phenotypic variability.

Diagnostic Studies.

- Noting observable signs and symptoms in the offspring is important since not all women are forthright about their prenatal alcohol exposure history
- Assessment of the child is often performed by a multidisciplinary team with input from a medical geneticist
- Height, weight, and head circumference are plotted on population-specific growth curves; watershed area is 10th percentile
- Facial dysmorphology examination includes use of guides for the subjective comparison of some variables (e.g., lip and philtrum features)

and precise anthropometric measurements of others (e.g., palpebral fissure length)
- Comprehensive **cognitive and developmental evaluation** is performed with use of standardized tests
- Neuroradiologic assessment may include EEG and brain MRI
- Key features in diagnostic criteria for FAS include the presence of CNS abnormalities, growth deficits, neurobehavioral impairment, and ≥ 2 facial abnormalities.

Morphologic Features in the CNS.
- Microcephaly
- Enlarged ventricles
- Agenesis of the corpus callosum
- Cerebellar hypoplasia

Differential Diagnosis. Facial dysmorphology may be caused by genetic disorders and other teratogens (hydantoin, valproate and toluene). A chromosome microarray study may be a first-tier test in individuals with a developmental delay. Karyotyping is used when the phenotypic features are strongly suggestive of a specific genetic disorder.

Treatment and Outcomes.
- There is no "safe level" of ethanol use during pregnancy; pregnant women are advised to abstain from ethanol use
- Early recognition of FAS is key to improved outcomes.
- **Behavioral sequelae** of the disease include higher unemployment rates and higher rates of illicit drug use and alcohol abuse.
- Treatment often involves input and consultation from pediatricians, physical therapists, psychiatrists, and special educators.

Physiology Correlation. Gastrulation is the embryonic differentiation of the blastula into the 3 germ layers: endoderm, mesoderm and ectoderm. The nervous system and neural crest arise from the ectoderm. Craniofacial cartilage and bone arise from neural crest. Ethanol affects multiple steps in **neural crest development**.

Pharmacology Correlation. In adults, the liver is the primary site of ethanol metabolism. In the first step, ethanol is oxidized to acetaldehyde, a known teratogen, which can cross the placental barrier. In the second phase, acetaldehyde gets broken down to acetate by acetaldehyde dehydrogenase. The primary enzyme in the first step of ethanol metabolism is alcohol dehydrogenase (ADH), which is present in negligible levels in the fetal liver. Ethanol is also oxidized to a lesser extent by the microsomal (cytochrome P450) ethanol oxidizing system, although its role in ethanol oxidation increases at higher ethanol concentrations. CYP2E1 is a cytochrome P450 enzyme that is upregulated by chronic alcohol use; it generates reactive oxygen species involved in many pathophysiologic conditions.

Vignette 2

> A 35-year-old man is involved in a ski accident in Colorado in the month of December. He returns home to Texas shortly thereafter, but begins to suffer from headaches. One day in January he tells his wife he cannot see, and she calls EMS.

Pathogenesis. Subdural hemorrhage (SDH) is a collection of blood in the space between the dura and the arachnoid. It is due to the tearing of stretched cortical bridging veins. **Acute subdural hemorrhage is usually related to a traumatic event** that causes a sudden accumulation of a large volume of blood. Bridging veins are more likely to tear in accidents causing a rapid acceleration. Epidural hematoma and diffuse axonal injury may exist concurrently with SDH. A high percentage of children dying from abuse have acute subdural hemorrhages. Chronic subdural hemorrhage can occur without a specific history of trauma, particularly in the elderly where brain atrophy causes enlargement of subarachnoid spaces. In some cases of chronic subdural hemorrhage associated with trauma, blood may slowly accumulate until compression of adjacent structures causes symptomatology.

Clinical Presentation. Acute subdural hemorrhage may cause immediate **loss of consciousness**. Symptoms of chronic subdural hemorrhage are more subtle; headache is one of the most common symptoms, and changes in cognitive ability may also occur. The patient in this vignette suffered visual loss from optic nerve compression.

Diagnostic Studies.
- Imaging studies (MRI and CT) are the key to diagnosis

Morphologic Features.
- Acute subdural hemorrhage: unilateral subdural blood over the fronto-parietal region.
- Skull fractures are present in 50% of acute subdural hemorrhage cases.
- A chronic subdural hemorrhage eventually forms an organized hematoma. Some organized chronic subdural hematomas show evidence of rebleeding.

Differential Diagnosis. The classic clinical history of an epidural hematoma is an immediate loss of consciousness followed by a temporary lucid interval with subsequent loss of consciousness. In the majority of epidural hematomas, bleeding originates from a torn meningeal artery in the temporal region.

Nervous and Special Senses

Treatment and Outcomes.
- For small subdural hemorrhages: careful observation and repeated head imaging
- For large hematomas: evacuation
- For chronic subdural hematomas: craniotomy for hematoma evacuation; alternative therapies include burr hole or twist drill drainage, followed by instillation of tissue plasminogen activator (tPA) to prevent recurrence

Physiology Correlation. Plasmin is a key fibrinolytic factor. It is a serine protease formed from its inactive precursor, plasminogen, by enzymes including urokinase and tissue plasminogen activator. Plasminogen is synthesized in the liver and circulates in peripheral blood.

Pharmacology Correlation. Recombinant **tissue plasminogen activator** is used to prevent recurrence of subdural hematoma because it selectively causes **local fibrinolysis** without systemically affecting hemostasis. It activates plasminogen that is bound to fibrin.

Vignette 3

A 43-year-old public health professor develops limb weakness and an ascending paralysis. She recently traveled to Haiti.

Pathogenesis. Guillain-Barré syndrome (GBS) is an immune-mediated, **demyelinating polyradiculoneuropathy**. Infection is believed to underlie the autoimmune process. Reported antecedent infections include bacteria (most commonly *Campylobacter jejuni*) and viruses: EBV, CMV, HIV and Zika virus.

Clinical Presentation. The patient in the vignette likely became infected with Zika virus in Haiti. Typically 2–4 weeks after an illness or vaccination, early symptoms of GBS occur. **Acroparesthesia** (numbness and tingling in fingers) and proximal muscle weakness of the lower extremities are followed by **ascending bilateral weakness**. Severe radicular back pain may occur. Autonomic symptoms include facial flushing and changes in heart rate and BP. Hyporeflexia or areflexia is usually noted on neurologic examination. Facial nerve involvement is common. Ultimately, respiration is compromised. Clinical variants exist and they can be distinguished from each other with electrophysiologic classification.

Clinical Disease Categories of GBS

Variant	Geographic Region	Notable Features	Basis
Acute inflammatory demyelinating polyneuropathy (AIDP)	Western countries	**Ascending paralysis**	Inflammatory demyelination
Miller Fisher syndrome (MFS)	Asia	Ophthalmoplegia, ataxia, and areflexia	Antibodies
Acute motor axonal neuropathy/acute motor and sensory axonal neuropathy (AMAN/AMSAN)	China/Japan/Mexico	Flaccid paralysis and areflexia without sensory loss	Axonal damage

Nervous and Special Senses

Diagnostic Studies.

- Lumbar puncture to evaluate CSF
- There is an **albuminocytologic dissociation** (increased protein, normal WBC count), but this finding may not be present until the second week
- Electrodiagnostic studies (electromyography and nerve conduction studies) may not be helpful during the early weeks of disease, but they can ultimately distinguish between subtypes
- Serum antibody testing to detect anti-GQ1b antibodies in MFS

Morphologic Features.

- Microscopic examination of a sural nerve biopsy shows perivascular myelin loss accompanied by a mononuclear infiltrate.

Differential Diagnosis. Diphtheria may involve the nervous system after initial pharyngeal infection, causing paralysis of the soft palate and oculomotor muscles before involving other muscle groups. *Corynebacterium diphtheria* causes a toxin-mediated, segmental demyelination with minimal inflammation. If sensory involvement is not present, myasthenia gravis and electrolyte disturbances are other diagnostic considerations. Diabetes mellitus is the most common cause of polyneuropathy.

Treatment and Outcomes.

- Supportive therapy: plasma exchange, IV immunoglobulin therapy, pain modulators, mechanical ventilation, anticoagulants, physical therapy and adaptive devices
- Half of patients experience prolonged disability but the majority recover
- Causes of death include infection, diffuse alveolar damage, and pulmonary embolism

Physiology Correlation. Two factors determine nerve conduction velocity: cell diameter and myelination. Loss of myelin results in current leakage across the cell membrane. Conduction block results from inadequate current reaching the fast Na^+ channels.

Pharmacology Correlation. **IV immunoglobulin therapy**, a blood product made from the pooled sera of multiple donors, has an immunomodulatory effect in patients with GBS. The therapy inhibits autoantibodies. Immediate, delayed and late adverse effects have been reported. There is a higher risk of an anaphylactic reaction in patients with IgA deficiency. Headache is the most common delayed adverse effect. Late reactions include renal failure and enteritis.

Nervous and Special Senses

Vignette 4

A 7-year-old boy presents to the doctor due to new onset of seizures. The mother reports that he has been falling down and "walking clumsily" for 6 months. He has also been performing poorly in school. The family history is uncertain due to adoption.

Pathogenesis. Juvenile Huntington disease (HD) (or Westphal variant) is an autosomal dominant disorder that results in degeneration of GABAergic neurons of the caudate nucleus. The gene, *HTT*, located on **chromosome 4**, codes for the **huntingtin protein**.

Clinical Presentation. Mean age is 40s, generally presenting with involuntary **choreiform movements**, mood/behavioral changes, and dementia. Juvenile HD (mean age <20) causes significant rigidity, hypokinesia and evidence of cerebellar involvement. Chorea may be absent. Learning difficulties and gait imbalance may present before seizures.

Diagnostic Studies.
- PCR to amplify a portion of the Huntington disease gene, in order to count the number of **triplet repeats of CAG** (cytosine-adenine-guanine)
- MRI (preferred imaging study) shows caudate head atrophy with relative enlargement of frontal horns causing a **boxcar configuration of the ventricles**

Morphologic Features.
- Gross examination of the brain: **bilateral atrophy of the caudate and putamen with ventricular enlargement**
- Microscopy: neuronal loss and astrocytosis in the neostriatal nuclei

Differential Diagnosis. Seizures are an important distinguishing feature in the differential diagnosis. Temporal lobe seizures are the presenting symptom in chorea-acanthocytosis, and generalized seizures occur in McLeod syndrome. Seizures are present only in the juvenile form of HD. Dentatorubral-pallidoluysian atrophy (DRPLA) is caused by a CAG repeat; it is difficult to clinically differentiate from HD but the affected gene is *ATN1*. Other heredodegenerative diseases might be a strong consideration in certain ethnic groups (e.g., Huntington disease-like 2 occurs in families with South African heritage, but there is no CAG expansion).

Treatment and Outcomes.
- Multidisciplinary care due to the decline in patient function
- There is no cure, and medical treatment is aimed at symptom management of chorea and mood disorder with GABA agonists, dopamine depleters, neuroleptics and antidepressants.
- Newer therapies include pallidotomy, fetal cell transplant and deep brain stimulation of the internal globus pallidus.
- Adult HD causes death in 14–15 years, while juvenile HD is more rapidly progressive, with death in <10 years.

Physiology Correlation. Gamma-aminobutyric acid (**GABA**) is an **inhibitory neurotransmitter**. Cell death of GABAergic neurons in the corpus striatum causes an increase of movement in HD.

Pharmacology Correlation. Tetrabenazine (TBZ) is a **dopamine-depleter** used to reduce the severity of chorea. One advantage to therapy with TBZ is that it does not cause tardive dyskinesia (repetitive involuntary movements such as darting of the tongue) caused by some of the typical neuroleptics.

Vignette 5

A 35-year-old man asks his fiancé to drive him to urgent care after 3 hours of dizziness, vomiting, and imbalance. Before he can see the doctor, he collapses in the parking lot.

Pathogenesis. Basilar artery occlusion (BAO) may cause a **posterior circulation stroke**. The more common etiologies include emboli from the heart, atherosclerosis, and arterial dissection (e.g., traumatic vertebral artery dissection). Rare causes include Behçet disease and neurosyphilis. Occlusion of the basilar artery may impact the brainstem, cerebellum, thalamus or occipital region.

Clinical Presentation. This subset of posterior circulation ischemia causes symptoms that are not typical of stroke, and for that reason, neurologic workup is often delayed. Prodromal symptoms include vertigo, nausea, headache, and neck pain. These symptoms are followed by a latent period that precedes the development of signs that prompt a workup for stroke. The predominating stroke symptomology is determined by the location of occlusion. For example, "**locked-in syndrome**" occurs when the pons becomes ischemic due to midbasilar occlusion; these patients are fully conscious but paralyzed. An infarct of the lower midbrain (as in vignette 5) may result in bilateral ataxia.

Diagnostic Studies.
- MRI is more sensitive than CT without contrast
- Early strokes, particularly in posterior circulation, may be diffusion-weighted imaging-negative
- An early negative MRI should not rule out stroke if neurologic deficits persist
- Cerebral angiogram is gold standard

Morphologic Features.
- Embolus: basilar artery emboli may cause bilateral cerebellar infarcts
- Atherosclerosis: plaque and superimposed thrombus
- Arterial dissection: hyalinized aneurysm wall with organizing thrombus

Differential Diagnosis. If hemiparesis is the predominating sign, an occlusion of the carotid circulation may be erroneously suspected. Basilar artery thrombosis needs to be identified and distinguished from peripheral vertigo of the inner ear; a bedside oculomotor examination (**h**ead **i**mpulse/**n**ystagmus/**t**est-of-**s**kew or HINTS) may be helpful to "rule in" peripheral vertigo before imaging changes would be expected for BAO. Vertigo can also be a feature of migraine headache; history, imaging and the evolution of the clinical course are helpful to make the distinction. Subarachnoid hemorrhage can be eliminated on the basis of imaging. Ruling out CNS infection requires CSF examination.

Treatment and Outcomes.
- IV tissue-type plasminogen activator (t-PA)
- Early endovascular treatment; recanalization improves outcome.
- Cases due to embolic etiology have a worse outcome.
- Mortality, which used to be 100%, is now reported to be as low as 30% in some series.

Physiology Correlation. Occlusion of the basilar artery is not always permanent. In some cases, possibly due to intrinsic fibrinolytic mechanisms, symptoms may resolve quickly leaving no neuroradiologic findings. In other cases, there may be clot fragmentation or migration. A transient ischemic attack is an ischemic event that resolves without evidence of tissue infarction; the term used to be defined by duration of signs and symptoms.

Pharmacology Correlation. Ischemic stroke is sometimes treated in the early stage with **tissue plasminogen activator for thrombolysis,** but its utility is limited and also controversial. When administered 3 hours (some say 4.5 hours) after stroke onset, the risk of hemorrhagic transformation increases, in part due to breakdown of the blood-brain barrier.

Vignette 6

A man in his 40s moves back to the United States from London and begins to feel depressed. He seeks help from a psychiatrist but withholds symptoms of memory loss. Following the onset of ataxia, he is referred to a neurologist. MRI reveals pulvinar sign. He dies 14 months later. Autopsy shows florid plaques.

Pathogenesis. Creutzfeldt-Jakob disease (CJD) is a **prion disease** resulting from a misfolded cellular protein. **Classic CJD** most often occurs sporadically (sCJD), but in 10% of cases, familial mutations of the gene encoding the major prion protein are present. Iatrogenic cases from contaminated neurosurgical instruments are rare due to modern sterilization protocols. **Variant CJD** (vCJD) occurs from foodborne exposure to the bovine spongiform encephalopathy (**BSE**) prion. Secondary infection can follow blood transfusions from donors with subclinical vCJD.

Clinical Presentation. There is a long latent phase of infection lasting decades. Sporadic CJD typically presents age 70s with rapid onset of **cognitive decline, ataxia**, and **myoclonus**; patients progress to akinetic mutism within weeks to a year. Familial CJD and vCJD present earlier in adulthood. Psychiatric symptoms often precede other manifestations in cases of vCJD, as seen in the vignette.

Diagnostic Studies.
- MRI findings of high signal on diffusion-weighted imaging in the caudate, putamen or cortex support the diagnosis; in vCJD, the **pulvinar sign** is the finding of bilateral hyperintensities in the pulvinar (posterior) thalamic nuclei
- Characteristic EEG findings are not always present; **periodic sharp wave complexes** are present in 50% of cases of sCJD but are not usually seen in vCJD
- Presence of **14-3-3 protein** in spinal fluid can also support the diagnosis
- Pathologic examination of brain biopsy or autopsy material is required for definitive diagnosis

Morphologic Features.
- Gross examination of the brain: Diffuse cerebral atrophy is rare due to rapid demise.
- Microscopy of brain tissue:
  - **Spongiform change** without inflammation in the cerebral cortex, putamen and thalamus
  - **Amyloid plaques** in vCJD

Nervous and Special Senses

Differential Diagnosis. CJD cases presenting with purely cognitive symptoms have to be distinguished from Alzheimer disease (AD). Both AD and CJD are caused by misfolded proteins. In AD there is abnormal folding of A_β peptide; in CJD there is abnormal folding of PrP^{sc}. Western blot allows identification of PrP^{SC}.

Treatment and Outcomes.

- No cure; treatment is palliative with opioids for pain and epilepsy medications for myoclonus.
- Most cases are fatal within a year; survival is minimally longer in vCJD.

Physiology Correlation. EEG measures voltage fluctuations in neural ionic currents. Action potentials depend on voltage-gated Na+ channels. Placement of electrodes on the skull allows a recording of the amplitude of the electrical signal generated by the current across neurons. **Periodic sharp wave complexes** are (EEG) findings that are seen in cases of CJD. Myoclonic jerks are associated with the sharp waveforms.

Pharmacology Correlation. Valproic acid (VPA) is an anticonvulsant sometimes used to treat the myoclonus associated with CJD. Hepatoxicity is one of the life-threatening adverse effects of sodium valproate. VPA undergoes biotransformation in the liver via multiple pathways including one in the mitochondria. There is an increased risk of liver failure due to VPA use in patients with mitochondrial disease due to *POLG* mutations, such as Alpers syndrome.

Nervous and Special Senses

Vignette 7

A 55-year-old man who was previously treated with radiation for head and neck cancer develops a new onset of headaches. He subsequently undergoes neuroimaging, and 2 parasagittal dural-based lesions are identified.

Pathogenesis. A **meningioma** is a tumor that arises from the **arachnoid cap cells** of the arachnoid membrane. These cells are present in high number in the arachnoid granulations and also in the tela choroidea of the ventricles although the location of the tumor is most often parasagittal. About 90% of the tumors have an intracranial location, 9% arise in the spine and the remaining cases arise in unusual extradural locations (e.g., scalp). Exposure to ionizing radiation confers the greatest risk. There may be familial susceptibilities to the effects of radiation. Type 2 neurofibromatosis (NF2) is the most common genetic association, and a meningioma in a patient age <40 leads to consideration of NF2, which is caused by a 22q deletion.

Clinical Presentation. Small, asymptomatic meningiomas may be found incidentally; symptomatic tumors may cause nonspecific findings of headache and paresis. The tumor is more common in middle-aged women. Meningiomas are more often solitary, but in cases secondary to radiation (vignette 7) and in NF2 cases, multiple tumors may exist.

Diagnostic Studies.
- MRI is imaging modality of choice
- On imaging, **CSF vascular cleft sign** points to the extra-axial location of the neoplasm
- A **dural tail** (thickening and enhancement of the dura) may be seen
- Intracranial meningioma does not typically invade the brain parenchyma but does cause adjacent edema

Morphologic Features.
- Variant meningiomas have a multitude of histologic patterns.
- Microscopic examination of a typical meningioma shows syncytial arrangements of cells with whorls. **Psammoma bodies** may be abundant. Nuclear vacuoles are common; nuclear atypia does not confer a worse prognosis, but necrosis does.

Differential Diagnosis. The varied microscopic appearance of the tumor and the tendency for metaplastic change makes microscopic diagnosis a challenge. Immunohistochemical positivity for epithelial membrane antigen (EMA) and vimentin is usual and S-100 staining is often negative. The meningeal location of the tumor and the attachment to the dura can help cinch a diagnosis, but if the tumor location is in the spine or the central pontine angle, other tumors bear consideration. In the spine, schwannomas occur more often in the lumbar region; meningiomas arise more often in the thoracic region.

Treatment and Outcomes.

- Typically benign, grade 1 tumors; according to 2017 WHO Classification of CNS Tumors, brain invasion increases grade to 2.
- Malignant meningiomas (grade 3) are more common in NF2 cases and in cases secondary to radiation.
- Surgical excision may be undertaken if excision would not cause significant morbidity; tumors may recur if excision is incomplete.

Physiology Correlation. Three protective layers of the CNS are the pia mater, the arachnoid, and the dura mater. The arachnoid villi are herniations of the arachnoid membrane that penetrate the dura and permit one-way flow of CSF into the venous sinuses of the brain, allowing metabolic by-products of the neurons and microglial cells to enter the peripheral circulation.

Pharmacology Correlation. Surgical excision and radiation therapy are the mainstay of meningioma treatment, and chemotherapeutic agents are typically not efficacious. Somatostatin receptors are present on some meningiomas. Recurrent meningioma has been treated with somatostatin analogs.

Vignette 8

A 28-year-old man is in his second month of treatment for tuberculosis when he begins to experience cognitive difficulty at work. A few weeks later, he has a generalized seizure at his office. A coworker drives him to the hospital, where a brain CT shows several ring-enhancing lesions.

Pathogenesis. **Toxoplasma encephalitis** is the most common CNS infection in HIV+ individuals who are not taking ART. It is often an index AIDS diagnosis. *Toxoplasma gondii* is an intracellular protozoan parasite; the organism can be spread iatrogenically by transplanted organ and whole blood transfusion. Another mode of infection is consumption of undercooked pork or mutton. Transplacental transmission and oral ingestion of feline oocysts also occur. Toxoplasma is ingested by a cat, enters the mucosa of the ileum, and following gamete fusion, oocysts are shed in the feces. Sporulation occurs in the external environment. Following oocyst ingestion by humans, sporozoites are released and transported by macrophages to organs, where asexual reproduction occurs in a nucleated cell. The trophozoites produce a protective membrane, resulting in a tissue cyst. A tissue cyst may contain more than a thousand organisms and may reach 200 μm in diameter. If the cyst ruptures, relapse occurs.

Clinical Presentation. Most infections are asymptomatic and self-limiting, and cysts can remain intact in the immunocompetent host. Reactivation of dormant infection can occur in the CNS in immunocompromised individuals, as with the man in the vignette who tested positive for HIV. Extracerebral infection is not as common. Patients may complain of nonspecific symptoms (headache, confusion, and fever) and focal neurologic symptoms. Seizures may also occur.

Diagnostic Studies.

- On imaging ≥1 **ring-enhancing lesions** are seen; other findings include edema and mass effect
- Frontal, basal ganglia, and parietal regions often involved
- Incidence of seropositivity is no higher in HIV+ population than general population
- IgG antibodies to *T. gondii* may be present
- Absence of antitoxoplasma antibodies does not rule out infection
- PCR testing of CSF is 100% specific but only about 50% sensitive for infection
- Brain biopsy is not always necessary for diagnosis
- CD4 counts are monitored throughout treatment; counts <100 cells/microliter increase risk of reactivation of toxoplasma infection

Morphologic Features of Brain Biopsy.
- Abscess
- Perivascular lymphocytic infiltrate
- Crescent-shaped tachyzoites (4–8 microns) free in the tissue and cysts encasing bradyzoites

Differential Diagnosis. Other ring-enhancing lesions include glioblastoma, large B-cell lymphoma, cerebral metastases, tuberculosis, and fungal infections. If the clinical suspicion of toxoplasmosis is high, a trial of therapy is offered with the expectation that symptoms will resolve in under a week and radiologic evidence of resolution will follow in a few weeks.

Treatment and Outcomes.
- Treatment of both AIDS and toxoplasmosis is necessary.
- Pyrimethamine and sulfadiazine are used for primary treatment of the parasite; neurologic response to treatment is expected within a week.
- Prophylaxis against reactivation.

Physiology Correlation. Toxoplasmosis infects astrocytes, neurons and microglia cells. Toxoplasma encephalitis activates astrocytes. Astrogliosis is a response to injury in the CNS that indicates a parenchymal injury has occurred. Astrocytic response to injury can cause an increase in the size and number of cells, but mitotic figures are almost never seen.

Pharmacology Correlation. Pyrimethamine and sulfadiazine nonselectively block folic acid metabolism. Treatment with folinic acid can improve folate stores.

Vignette 9

A 40-year-old man begins to have attacks of dizziness that cause him to lie down in bed. The attacks are accompanied by nausea and vomiting. When he seeks help from his doctor, he reports that he has also been experiencing episodic fluctuations in hearing, as well as ringing in the right ear.

Pathogenesis. Ménière's disease (MD) is a peripheral vestibular disorder that causes chronic vertigo. The pathogenesis is still not completely elucidated, but recent theories center around swelling of the endolymph compartment that creates pressure in the inner ear. While there is an association between **endolymph hydrops** and MD, it is inconstant and possibly only correlative.

Clinical Presentation. The disease most often presents at age 40-60 years. Classic features include episodes of **vertigo**, nausea, aural fullness, **tinnitus**, and **asymmetrical hearing loss**. The hearing loss is initially in low frequencies and progresses to high frequencies. Hearing loss worsens with each episode, and severe unilateral hearing loss ultimately occurs over time in most cases.

Diagnostic Studies.
- Diagnosis rests on clinical symptoms and audiometric testing
- **Pure tone audiogram** to evaluate hearing; MD often causes **a low frequency hearing loss**
- Ancillary studies to rule out other conditions
- Microscopic examination of tissue is not part of clinical diagnostic process

Morphologic Features of temporal bone [microscopic findings from autopsy series].
- Hair cell loss
- Basement membrane thickening
- Perivascular microvascular damage

Differential Diagnosis. In patients with unilateral hearing loss, it is important to exclude cerebellopontine angle tumor and acoustic neuroma with imaging (MRI). The symptoms of hearing loss, vertigo and tinnitus may also occur with anterior inferior cerebellar artery stroke, but other localizing signs such as ataxia would be expected. Viral infection (e.g., mumps) can cause unilateral or bilateral hearing loss. The vertigo of benign paroxysmal positional vertigo can be triggered with sudden head motion. Vestibular migraine can also cause vertigo.

Nervous and Special Senses

Treatment and Outcomes.
- No cure; treatment is aimed at controlling symptoms.
- Salt restriction and diuretics are beneficial.
- Intratympanic gentamicin therapy improves vertigo but hearing loss is an adverse effect.

Physiology Correlation. Equilibrium is maintained by the vestibular system in the inner ear. Head movements cause a flow of endolymph in the semicircular canals. Endolymph is a potassium-rich fluid that fills the membranous labyrinth.

Pharmacology Correlation. Gentamicin and streptomycin can cause injury to vestibular hair cells, and in fact, it is the vestibulotoxic effects that are sought in treatment of the disease. Nonetheless, both drugs can cause permanent hearing loss.

Vignette 10

After a brief viral illness, a 16-year-old girl begins to suffer from episodes of tachycardia, lightheadedness, and brain fog. The symptoms persist for months, and her pediatrician refers her to a cardiologist. A tilt table test is performed.

Pathogenesis. Postural orthostatic tachycardia syndrome (POTS) (also known as soldier's heart and chronic orthostatic intolerance) is a disorder of the autonomic nervous system. The pathogenesis is not entirely understood. Genetic factors and infection may play a role. In some cases it follows an infectious illness. Topics of interest include the role of abnormalities of mast cell activation, leg blood flow, increased release and/or decreased clearance of epinephrine, and atypical blood volume regulation.

Clinical Presentation. POTS can present at any age but it is more common in reproductive age women. There is often a preceding history of viral illness, as in the vignette. **Orthostatic intolerance** manifests as an increase in heart rate accompanied by other bothersome symptoms upon standing. In most patients, hyperadrenergic symptoms (headache, dizziness, tremulousness) predominate. GI complaints are common: nausea and vomiting (most common) followed by abdominal pain, early satiety, and bloating. Symptoms of fatigue, exercise intolerance, and near-syncope may cause significant disability.

Diagnostic Studies.
- Orthostatic vital signs (measurement of heart rate and BP in supine and standing position) to look for increased heart rate >30 bpm (>40 bpm if age <18) in first 10 minutes of standing in the absence of a significant decrease in BP
- Assessment of cardiac function via examination and possibly by echocardiography
- Quantitative sudomotor axon reflex testing to detect autonomic dysfunction.
- Exercise capacity assessment may be offered during follow-up

Morphologic Features.
- A POTS diagnosis is not made based on tissue changes that can be observed grossly or with a microscope
- Preliminary research indicates that small fiber neuropathy has been identified in skin biopsies in a subset of patients

Differential Diagnosis. Since dysautonomia is a clinical diagnosis of exclusion, other etiologies for the symptoms need to be ruled out (e.g., arrhythmia

Nervous and Special Senses

or structural heart disease). Dysautonomia can occur secondary to other medical conditions, for example, multiple sclerosis. Sometimes when the features of dysautonomia are not recognized, attention to certain specific symptoms that accompany POTS (e.g., depression) may delay diagnosis of POTS. Somatization disorders may be considered before POTS if orthostatic vital signs are not part of the workup. Fainting is a significant feature of another form of dysautonomia, neurocardiogenic syncope (also known as vasovagal syncope); POTS patients may only feel lightheaded and never actually faint (near-syncope).

Treatment and Outcomes.

- Medical treatment approaches include fludrocortisone (to increase blood volume), beta-blockers (to control heart rate) and cholinesterase inhibitors.

- Some patients improve with medical treatment and lifestyle changes including diet modification (increased water intake, decreased salt intake) and exercise training. For others the condition worsens with time.

- Around 25% of those with POTS are disabled by the condition.

Physiology Correlation. The heart rate normally increases when a person stands to compensate for the fall in plasma volume that occurs upon standing. The shift in blood flow to the lower extremities causes a decrease in thoracic venous blood volume. Decreased right ventricular preload leads to a decline in stroke volume by the Frank-Starling mechanism. Baroreceptors respond to the decrease in systemic arterial pressure, and autonomic neurons in the medulla respond by increasing sympathetic outflow and decreasing parasympathetic outflow. Vasoconstriction, tachycardia and positive inotropy ensue. Epinephrine stimulates the beta receptors of the sinoatrial node cells.

Pharmacology Correlation. Propanolol is a nonselective beta-adrenergic blocking agent. Beta-1 receptors are present in the heart, and beta-2 receptors are present in gland cells and smooth muscle (hence the drug exacerbates asthma). The effects of propranolol on the heart are greater during higher demand, such as exercise. **Propanolol is a negative inotrope**.

Test What You Have Learned

1. A 78-year-old woman is found unconscious lying on the cement steps going up to her house. She is taken to the local ED, where she is noted to be unresponsive. She also has a large bruise on her forehead. This patient's condition is most likely related to which of the following?

   A. Agenesis of the corpus callosum

   B. Basilar artery occlusion

   C. Bilateral atrophy of caudate and putamen

   D. Ring-enhancing lesion of basal ganglia

   E. Spongiform change in cerebral cortex, putamen, and thalamus

   F. Sural nerve shows perivascular myelin loss

   G. Tearing of cortical bridging veins

2. A 54-year-old woman undergoes MRI of the brain for evaluation of chronic headaches that have been worsening in severity for the last several years. The MRI demonstrates a 3 cm round mass on the lateral surface of the cerebral cortex. Imaging also reveals a CSF vascular cleft sign between the mass and the underlying lateral surface of the cerebral cortex. If the mass recurs after resection, which of the following therapies would be the most helpful?

   A. Fludrocortisone

   B. Intratympanic gentamicin

   C. IV immunoglobulin therapy

   D. IV tissue-type plasminogen activator

   E. Pyrimethamine and sulfadiazine

   F. Somatostatin analogs

   G. Tetrabenazine

3. A 68-year-old woman who, until 2 years ago, had appeared normal for her age undergoes a rapidly progressive intellectual decline. Her coordination deteriorates to the point that she cannot walk and she becomes immobile. About 2 years after the neurologic symptoms started, she stops speaking. Her difficulties are most likely to be related to which of the following molecules?

    A. Alcohol
    B. Anti-CQ1b
    C. ATN1
    D. CYP2E1
    E. Gaba-aminobutyric acid
    F. PrP^{sc}

4. During a trip to Mexico, a 7-year-old boy develops a low-grade fever with rash and joint pain. Two weeks later the boy experiences first tingling and pain in his legs, and then progressive leg weakness. Infection with which of the following would have been most likely to have contributed to the boy's physical problems?

    A. *Campylobacter jejuni*
    B. HIV
    C. Prion
    D. Syphilis
    E. *Toxoplasma gondii*
    F. Zika virus

5. A 35-year-old woman has been experiencing mood swings for 5 years. She has been more forgetful lately, and her family thinks her judgement is beginning to be impaired. Other family members have had similar symptoms. Which of the following would be most likely to establish the patient's diagnosis?

    A. "Albuminocytology" on lumbar puncture
    B. Chromosome microarray study
    C. CSF vascular cleft sign
    D. Dural tail
    E. Head circumference <10 percentile
    F. PCR to look for triple repeats

Answers: 1. (G), 2. (F), 3. (F), 4. (F), 5. (F)

CHAPTER 3

Musculoskeletal System

Checklist of Processes Within This System

Developmental and Inherited Disorders
- ❑ Achondroplasia
- ❑ Osteogenesis imperfecta
- ❑ Duchenne muscular dystrophy
- ❑ Becker muscular dystrophy
- ❑ Syndactyly
- ❑ VACTERL association

Infections
- ❑ Osteomyelitis
- ❑ Lyme disease
- ❑ Suppurative arthritis
- ❑ Pott disease
- ❑ *Clostridium*

Inflammatory Diseases
- ❑ Gout
- ❑ Pseudogout
- ❑ Osteoarthritis

Diseases of the Immune System
- ❑ Rheumatoid arthritis
- ❑ Seronegative spondylarthropathies
- ❑ Inflammatory myopathies
- ❑ Myasthenia gravis
- ❑ Lambert-Eaton syndrome

Trauma
- ❑ Crush injuries
- ❑ Compartment syndrome

System-Specific Diseases
- ❑ Paget disease
- ❑ Metabolic disorders: osteitis fibrosa cystica; rickets; osteomalacia; osteoporosis

Tumors
- ❑ Osteoid osteoma
- ❑ Osteoblastoma
- ❑ Osteoma
- ❑ Giant cell tumor of bone
- ❑ Osteosarcoma
- ❑ Chondrosarcoma
- ❑ Ewing sarcoma
- ❑ Lipoma
- ❑ Liposarcoma
- ❑ Fibrosarcoma
- ❑ Undifferentiated pleomorphic sarcoma
- ❑ Leiomyoma
- ❑ Leiomyosarcoma
- ❑ Synovial sarcoma
- ❑ Alveolar rhabdomyosarcoma

Representative Diseases

What follows are clinical vignettes for 10 select diseases within this organ system. First, read the vignette and try to identify the condition. Then, move on to read integrated information on each disease.

Vignette 1

A 5-year-old girl is taken to the pediatrician for evaluation of short stature. On physical exam she has multiple lower extremity bruises and bluish scleral discoloration. Dental exam reveals multiple cavities. Audiological evaluation reveals a conductive hearing loss. Radiographic skeletal survey reveals healed right seventh rib and right humerus fractures and a healing left midshaft clavicle fracture. The physician does not suspect child abuse.

Diagnosis? _____

Vignette 2

A 47-year-old man presents to his primary doctor with 2 weeks of fever, headache, and muscle aches. He also has noted a nonpruritic erythematous rash in the right groin. The rash has been enlarging for the past week, with new areas of clearing resulting in concentric rings of erythema. The patient is a Boy Scout leader and recently returned from a camping trip in Connecticut.

Diagnosis? _____

Vignette 3

A 45-year-old man presents to urgent care with 2 days of left knee pain, swelling, and erythema without recent trauma. He is afebrile. White blood cell count, ESR, and CRP are mildly elevated. Knee x-ray shows a large joint effusion but is otherwise normal. On further questioning he reports a similar episode of acute onset joint pain and swelling involving the right 1st metatarsophalangeal joint 3 years ago.

Diagnosis? _____

Vignette 4

A 62-year-old woman presents with chronic left hip pain that is worse with activity. She has no history of trauma or malignancy. Left hip x-ray shows a bowing deformity of the proximal left femur, with expansion of the proximal femoral medullary space and proximal femoral cortical thickening. Lab evaluation reveals elevated alkaline phosphatase but normal serum calcium and phosphate. A nuclear medicine bone scan is performed to evaluate for other potential sites of involvement.

Diagnosis? _____

Musculoskeletal

Vignette 5

A 22-month-old child presents with abnormal bowing of the legs and difficulty walking. He was exclusively breastfed until age 12 months. He lives in a cold climate with limited exposure to direct sunlight. Physical exam reveals bowlegs, wrist soft tissue swelling, and open anterior fontanelle. Wrist x-ray shows osteopenia with cupping and fraying of the distal radial metaphyses.

Diagnosis? _____

Vignette 6

A 57-year-old woman presents with a red, scaly, itchy rash along the dorsal surface of the metacarpophalangeal (MCP) and interphalangeal (IP) joints of the hands. The rash worsens with sun exposure and her fingertips become painful and purplish on exposure to cold temperatures. She also complains of recent bilateral thigh pain and difficulty standing from a sitting position.

Diagnosis? _____

Vignette 7

A 60-year-old man arrives at the ED with an acute onset left distal thigh pain. He has had a deep, dull, achy pain at this same site for the past year. The acute pain started after minimal trauma while stumbling off a curb. There is no other acute trauma. Left knee x-rays show a 7 cm intramedullary lucent lesion in the distal femur with irregular "rings-and-arcs" type matrix mineralization. The bone cortex adjacent to the lesion is destroyed and there is aggressive-appearing periosteal reaction.

Diagnosis? _____

Vignette 8

A 37-year-old man presents with lower back pain. He complains of stiffness in his axial spine that usually improves over the course of the morning with activity. X-ray of the lumbar spine is normal, while x-ray of the sacroiliac joints shows bilateral abnormality including irregular joint space widening with bone erosions and subchondral sclerosis. HLA-B27 is positive.

Diagnosis? _____

Musculoskeletal

Vignette 9

An 18-year-old man presents with a painless, enlarging right thigh soft tissue mass for 3 months. He reports no history of prior thigh trauma. Physical exam reveals a hard, nonmobile and noncompressible soft tissue mass. Plain x-ray shows a noncalcified soft tissue mass measuring 10 cm.

Diagnosis? _____

Vignette 10

A 21-year-old man arrives at the ED from a construction site. His right lower extremity was trapped under a metal beam for 1 hour prior to extrication. There is evidence of blunt trauma to the right thigh, but there is no obvious penetrating injury. Lab evaluation reveals hyperkalemia and severe elevation of creatine kinase (CK).

Diagnosis? _____

Musculoskeletal

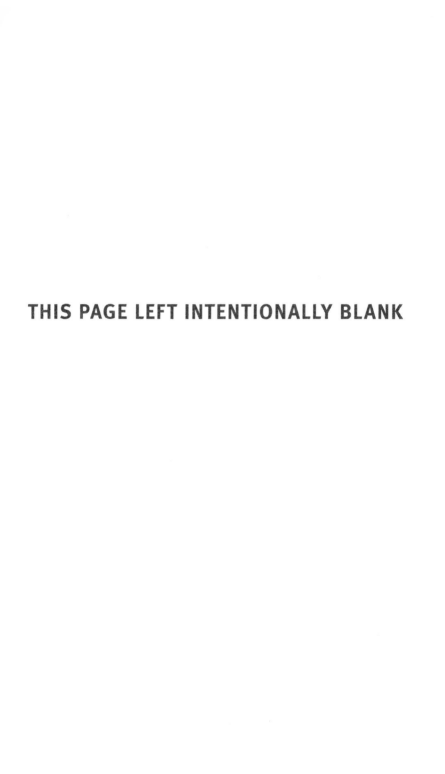
THIS PAGE LEFT INTENTIONALLY BLANK

Vignette 1

A 5-year-old girl presents to the pediatrician for evaluation of short stature. On physical exam she has multiple lower extremity bruises and bluish scleral discoloration. Dental exam reveals multiple cavities. Audiological evaluation reveals a conductive hearing loss. Radiographic skeletal survey reveals healed right seventh rib and right humerus fractures and a healing left midshaft clavicle fracture. The physician does not suspect child abuse.

Pathogenesis. **Osteogenesis imperfecta** (OI)—also called brittle bone disease, blue sclera syndrome, or fragile bone disease—is a genetic defect of connective disease. Most cases have autosomal dominant inheritance. There is a defect in the quantity or quality of type I collagen, which is an important component of bone, tendons, ligaments, and sclera. Nine types of OI have been categorized; type I is the mildest and type II is the most severe. Mutations in the *COL1A1* and *COL1A2* genes occur in >90% of cases. Most cases of type II OI are due to new gene mutations rather than inherited disease. The bones are osteopenic, leading to frequent fractures. Other clinical features depend on the specific gene mutation and include dental disease, hearing loss, and muscle weakness.

Clinical Presentation. The most severe form of OI (type II) is lethal in utero or early infancy. Patients with the most common and mildest form of OI (type I) have weakened bones with frequent fractures, premature hearing loss, and normal/near-normal stature.

Diagnostic Studies.
- History and physical exam diagnostic in most cases
- Radiographic skeletal survey to evaluate for clinically occult fractures
- DEXA scan to determine bone mineral density
- Genetic testing performed for genetic counseling

Morphologic Features.
- Gross examination: Bones have a thin, slender shape with thin cortices and decreased medullary cancellous bone; fractures at multiple stages of healing can be seen.
- Microscopy: Trabeculae are diminished with poorly developed Haversian systems and wide osteoid seams; collagen fibers are attenuated and appear in a random distribution.

Differential Diagnosis. Child abuse must be considered in any child who has multiple fractures in different stages of healing. Fractures of the skull, sternum, scapulae, posterior ribs and metaphysical corners are concerning for nonaccidental trauma (child abuse). A metabolic disorder such as rickets is also a consideration in any osteopenic child with multiple fractures.

Treatment and Outcomes.

- Ambulation aids, including braces and wheelchairs
- Orthopedic surgery referral to address bony deformities
- Bisphosphonates to increase bone density and decrease pathologic fractures

Physiology Correlation.

There are 4 types of collagen:

- Type I: primary collagen type in bone and tendons; is deficient or defective in OI
- Type II: found in cartilage
- Type III: found in skin and blood vessels; is defective in some forms of Ehlers-Danlos syndrome
- Type IV collagen: primary type in basement membranes
  - Mutations in the collagen IV genes cause Alport syndrome
  - In Goodpasture syndrome, autoantibodies form against type IV collagen present in basement membranes of pulmonary alveoli and renal glomeruli.

Pharmacology Correlation. Bisphosphonates are commonly used to treat OI, osteoporosis, and Paget disease. Known complications of bisphosphonates are esophagitis, insufficiency fractures of the proximal femurs, and osteonecrosis of the mandible.

Musculoskeletal

Vignette 2

A 47-year-old man presents to his primary doctor with 2 weeks of fever, headache, and muscle aches. He also has noted a nonpruritic erythematous rash in the right groin. The rash has been enlarging for the past week, with new areas of clearing resulting in concentric rings of erythema. The patient is a Boy Scout leader and recently returned from a camping trip in Connecticut.

Pathogenesis. **Lyme disease** is a multisystem inflammatory disease caused by the bite of the infected Ixodes tick. It results in infection with spirochetes of the *Borrelia* genus. *Borrelia burgdorferi* is the most common in the United States. Tick exposure in an endemic region is critical to diagnosis. In the United States, endemic areas include New England, Mid-Atlantic, and North Central states. Symptoms result from direct bacterial organ involvement and from the resultant immune response.

Clinical Presentation. Lyme has 3 stages: early localized stage (1 wk to 1 mo), early disseminated stage (several weeks to months), and late persistent stage (months to years). Findings of the early localized stage are typically the classic erythema migrans rash and inflammatory symptoms such as fever, weakness, headache, and myalgias. Findings of the early disseminated and late persistent stages may be cardiac and central nervous system effects, including AV block. Classic neurologic complications include meningitis and cranial nerve palsies, especially Bell's palsy. Arthritis is a common feature of the late persistent stage.

Diagnostic Studies.

- Classic erythema migrans rash acquired in an endemic region is sufficient for diagnosis
- Lab evaluation is based on a 2-tiered serologic test including ELISA and Western blot
- Serologic testing should not be performed without good exposure history (high false-positive rate)
- Lumbar puncture and joint aspiration needed with meningeal symptoms or monoarthritis

Morphologic Features.

- Skin biopsy shows a superficial and deep perivascular lymphocytic infiltrate; plasma cells are seen at the periphery of the skin lesion, and eosinophils in the center.

Musculoskeletal

Differential Diagnosis. The symptoms in each stage of Lyme disease have their own differential diagnosis. In the early localized stage, the differential for nonspecific inflammatory likely symptoms with joint pain includes an inflammatory arthritis such as rheumatoid arthritis or a seronegative spondyloarthropathy. Collagen vascular diseases such as lupus can have a similar presentation with multisystem involvement.

Treatment and Outcomes.

- Doxycycline (first-line treatment) for early localized disease
- Disease does not produce immunity; reinfection is possible
- Antibiotic therapy typically results in a cure

Physiology Correlation. Lyme carditis is associated with heart block. Heart block is diagnosed with 12-lead EKG and continuous holder monitoring. First-degree AV block is the mildest form and associated with an increased PR interval (>0.2 seconds). PR interval is measured from the beginning of the P wave to the beginning of the QRS complex. Heart block in Lyme disease can progress rapidly from first to third degree or complete heart block, where there is complete dissociation of electrical impulses between the atria and ventricles. Third-degree heart block can be fatal if untreated.

Pharmacology Correlation. Doxycycline is a tetracycline-class antibiotic commonly prescribed to treat Lyme. Doxycycline use is commonly associated with photosensitivity and is a known cause of pill-esophagitis. Patients should limit sun exposure and consume this medication with large amounts of water, in an upright position.

Musculoskeletal

Vignette 3

A 45-year-old man presents to urgent care with 2 days of left knee pain, swelling, and erythema without recent trauma. He is afebrile. White blood cell count, ESR, and CRP are mildly elevated. Knee x-ray shows a large joint effusion but is otherwise normal. On further questioning he reports a similar episode of acute onset joint pain and swelling involving the right 1st metatarsophalangeal joint 3 years ago.

Pathogenesis. Gout is an inflammatory arthritis caused by monosodium urate (MSU) monohydrate crystals. Acute gout is an acute inflammatory response to MSU crystal deposition in joints or soft tissue. Chronic tophaceous gout occurs with long-standing hyperuricemia. Hyperuricemia may occur due to overproduction or undersecretion. Risk factors for gout include advanced age, family history, obesity, and certain drugs including diuretics and chemotherapy. Triggers include alcoholic beverages and foods rich in purines (e.g., red meat).

Clinical Presentation. Gout tends to occur after decade 4 and is much more common in men than women. The disease has distinct phases. Acute gout is typically monoarticular, with the first metatarsophalangeal joint (podagra) most commonly affected with swelling, warmth, erythema and pain. The pain may be worse at night. A long asymptomatic phase is typical between acute attacks. Chronic tophaceous gout ultimately develops, causing damage to joints and forming periarticular cutaneous deposits of uric acid. These painful, yellowish subcutaneous nodules are called *tophi* (singular, ***tophus***); they commonly form along extensor surfaces and at the fingertips and ears.

Diagnostic Studies.

- Early in disease, x-ray shows joint effusion, and joint aspiration shows MSU crystals (needle-shaped and negatively birefringent)
- Imaging is most helpful in chronic gout when soft tissue tophi are visible; bone lesions are erosive and have overhanging edges
- Lab investigation shows increased serum uric acid levels

Morphologic Features.

Microscopy of joint aspirate: MSU crystals are needle-shaped and negatively birefringent under polarized light microscopy.

- Microscopy of skin biopsy: palisaded histiocytes surrounding crystals

Differential Diagnosis. Septic arthritis (joint infection) must be excluded in any case of acute monoarticular arthritis with synovial fluid examination. In infection, there is a fluid WBC >50,000/mcL. Other crystal deposition diseases, such as pseudogout (calcium pyrophosphate crystal deposition disease or CPCDD), can be distinguished from gout by synovial crystal analysis. CPCDD is characterized by rhomboid-shaped, positively birefringent crystals. Rheumatoid arthritis (RA) is a common noninfectious inflammatory arthritis. Joint involvement in RA is more commonly bilateral and symmetric compared to gout. Osteoarthritis (OA) is a noninflammatory arthritis that can have associated knee pain, swelling, and joint effusion. OA can be distinguished from its inflammatory counterparts by the pattern of joint involvement and synovial fluid analysis.

Treatment and Outcomes.

- NSAIDs, colchicine, and steroids for acute gout (usually resolves within several days of treatment)
- Lifestyle changes: weight loss and avoidance of dietary triggers
- Treatment of hyperuricemia with xanthine oxidase inhibitors (e.g., allopurinol) and uricosuric agents (e.g., probenecid)

Physiology Correlation. DNA and RNA are metabolized to hypoxanthine and guanine, respectively. These metabolites are both converted to xanthine, which is an immediate precursor to uric acid. Excessive uric acid accumulation causes the symptoms of gout. Uric acid is normally successfully excreted in the kidneys. Hyperuricemia results when there is an excess in the nucleic acid breakdown products, such as with the consumption of large amounts of red meat or with certain malignancies such as leukemia where there is high cell turnover. Hyperuricemia can also result from impaired renal clearance of uric acid. In particular, the metabolites of alcohol compete with uric acid in the kidneys.

Pharmacology Correlation. Allopurinol dosage is titrated to attain serum uric acid levels of <6 mg/dL. Interruption of therapy may cause an acute attack of gout. Side effects of the drug include abdominal pain, nausea and vomiting. Fatal hypersensitivity reactions are rare.

Musculoskeletal

Vignette 4

A 62-year-old woman presents with chronic left hip pain that is worse with activity. She has no history of trauma or malignancy. Left hip x-ray shows a bowing deformity of the proximal left femur, with expansion of the proximal femoral medullary space and proximal femoral cortical thickening. Lab evaluation reveals elevated alkaline phosphatase but normal serum calcium and phosphate. A nuclear medicine bone scan is performed to evaluate for other potential sites of involvement.

Pathogenesis. Paget disease of the bone is a localized idiopathic disorder of abnormal bone remodeling, resulting in mechanically weaker bone. Weakened pagetic bone can result in bowing deformities and pathologic fractures. Osteoarthritis results when Paget disease occurs near a joint. Enlarged pagetic bone can compress adjacent anatomic structures, like cranial nerves, when there is skull base involvement. Sarcomatous degeneration of pagetic bone is a feared complication that occurs in <1% of cases.

Clinical Presentation. Paget disease most commonly affects the bones of the skull, spine, pelvis and proximal femurs. Localized chronic pain and deformity occur as a result of direct bone involvement or from secondary causes, such as nerve compression or osteoarthritis of an involved joint. Patients can present with acute pain after pathologic fracture.

Diagnostic Studies.
- Elevated serum alkaline phosphatase
- X-ray of symptomatic sites shows typical cortical and medullary thickening of bone with bowing deformities and possible pathologic fractures
- Nuclear medicine bone scan is performed at diagnosis to evaluate for multifocal disease

Morphologic Features.
Microscopic features of bone vary depending on the stage of disease:
- Osteolysis early: numerous osteoclasts
- Mixed osteolytic-osteoblastic phase: numerous osteoblasts; mosaic or "jigsaw" pattern
- Late osteosclerotic phase: poorly mineralized new bone formation

Differential Diagnosis. Common differential diagnoses for chronic focal bone pain and deformity include old poorly healed fracture, chronic bone infection and both benign and malignant bone tumors. The clinical history and imaging appearance help differentiate these entities from Paget disease.

Musculoskeletal

Treatment and Outcomes.

- NSAIDs for control of bone pain and bisphosphonates to limit bone turnover
- Orthopedic-assist devices and surgery for primary bone deformities or secondary complications such as osteoarthritis and pathologic fracture

Physiology Correlation. Paget disease results in aggressive localized osteoclastic activity in bone followed by disorganized osteoblastic repair of bone. A nuclear medicine bone scan shows increased regions of tracer uptake at sites of aggressive osteoblastic activity. In the early phase of Paget, the lytic osteoclastic process can appear photopenic on a bone scan with relatively decreased tracer uptake compared to the adjacent normal bone.

Pharmacology Correlation. NSAIDs are used for pain control in Paget. Traditional NSAIDs block both cyclooxygenase (COX)-1 and cyclooxygenase (COX)-2 enzymes. COX-1 contributes to the formation of a protective lining, shielding the stomach from acid injury. COX-2 is the enzyme involved in the inflammatory cascade that results in pain. Selective COX-2 inhibitors do not interfere with the protective effect of COX-1 and are less likely to cause GI bleeding, compared to traditional NSAIDs.

Musculoskeletal

Vignette 5

A 22-month-old child presents with abnormal bowing of the legs and difficulty walking. He was exclusively breastfed until age 12 months. He lives in a cold climate with limited exposure to direct sunlight. Physical exam reveals bowlegs, wrist soft tissue swelling, and open anterior fontanelle. Wrist x-ray shows osteopenia with cupping and fraying of the distal radial metaphyses.

Pathogenesis. Rickets results from abnormal mineralization of osteoid in the growing skeleton, i.e., poorly mineralized osteoid leads to weakened bones. It can result from a deficiency of vitamin D. Most commonly, the vitamin D deficiency results from nutritional or environmental factors. Infants who are exclusively breastfed are at risk, as human milk contains minimal vitamin D. Increased melanin concentration in dark skinned individuals blocks the UV light needed to form vitamin D. Rickets can also be a result of a genetic disorder resulting in impaired vitamin D metabolism or impaired end-organ response to vitamin D.

Clinical Presentation. General hypotonia is common. Thinning/softening of skull bones (craniotabes) is seen in infants. Thickening of the skull is seen in older children with rickets, resulting in frontal bossing and delayed closure of the anterior fontanelle. Bowlegs or knock-knees (genu varum or genu valgum, respectively) is common. Build-up of nonossified cartilage at the metaphases of long bones results in focal soft tissue swelling, which is commonly seen at the wrists and knees. This same process results in expansion of the anterior ribs at the costochondral junctions (referred to as the *rachitic rosary*).

Diagnostic Studies.
- Low serum calcium, serum phosphorus, calcidiol, calcitriol
- Low urinary calcium
- High parathyroid hormone, alkaline phosphatase, and urinary phosphorus
- X-ray of rapidly growing regions such as wrists and knees show the classic cupping, fraying, and splaying of the metaphases and widening of growth plates

Morphologic Features.

Microscopic examination of bone:
- **Unmineralized osteoid tissue**
- Thickened growth plate on the metaphyseal side

Differential Diagnosis. Bowing deformities of the lower extremities can be seen with skeletal dysplasias, like achondroplasia, and in Blount disease in children. These are distinguished from rickets by normal serum chemistry. Osteogenesis imperfecta results in weak bones with bowing deformities, due to a defect in type 1 collagen.

Treatment and Outcomes.

- Vitamin D, calcium and phosphorus supplementation for nutritional rickets
- Parent counseling about risk factors like sun exposure and appropriate diet
- Orthopedic consultation for braces or possible surgical correction of bony deformities

Physiology Correlation. The active form of vitamin D is formed through a series of metabolic steps involving the skin, the liver, and the kidney. While the active form of vitamin D is calcitriol, it is serum calcidiol that is measured to evaluate vitamin D status. Calcitriol has a short half-life and exists at a much lower concentration than calcidiol.

Pharmacology Correlation. Phenytoin is a commonly prescribed seizure medication that increases risk of osteomalacia due to inhibition of calcium absorption in the small intestine.

Musculoskeletal

Vignette 6

A 57-year-old woman presents with a red, scaly, itchy rash along the dorsal surface of the metacarpophalangeal (MCP) and interphalangeal (IP) joints of the hands. The rash worsens with sun exposure and her fingertips become painful and purplish on exposure to cold temperatures. She also complains of recent bilateral thigh pain and difficulty standing from a sitting position.

Pathogenesis. Dermatomyositis (DM) is an immune-mediated necrotizing myopathy with characteristic dermatologic changes. When this myopathy exists without cutaneous findings, the term *polymyositis* is used. Malignancy (including lung, ovarian, gastric and colorectal) is present in up to 25% of patients with DM. Other immunologic triggers associated with the myositis-specific autoantibodies include certain infections (e.g., enterovirus) and drugs (e.g., statins).

Clinical Presentation. Cutaneous changes may occur years before noticeable muscle weakness. Characteristic cutaneous findings of DM include a periorbital heliotrope rash and Gottron papules along the extensor surface of the MCP and IP joints. Muscle injury results in muscle weakness, abnormal muscle enzyme levels (creatine kinase [CK]), and abnormal electromyography (EMG). Symmetric proximal muscle weakness in DM results in difficulty getting out of a chair, climbing steps, or combing hair. Extramuscular disease—including interstitial lung disease and cardiac involvement with rhythm abnormalities and conduction defects—significantly contributes to morbidity and mortality.

Diagnostic Studies.
- Elevated CK levels indicative of muscle injury
- Radiographs can show soft tissue calcification in a "lace-like" or "sheet-like" distribution
- MRI shows muscle edema at sites of muscle inflammation and helps guide muscle biopsy
- Electromyographic (EMG) testing confirms a myopathic process
- CT of the chest, abdomen and pelvis to evaluate for malignancy

Morphologic Features.
- Skin biopsy of erythematous lesions shows epidermal atrophy with vacuolization of the basal layer and a mild perivascular lymphocytic infiltrate.
- Gottron's papules show acanthosis.
- Muscle biopsy shows muscle fiber necrosis and an inflammatory infiltrate.

Differential Diagnosis. Laboratory investigation may be necessary to distinguish DM from its histologic lookalike, system lupus erythematosus, especially in cases where the skin changes of DM precede muscle weakness. In cases where muscle weakness predominates, the differential includes various metabolic (inherited metabolic disorders with adult onset), endocrine (hyperthyroid myopathy), infectious, and drug- or toxin-related processes.

Treatment and Outcomes.

- High-dose corticosteroids (first-line treatment)
- Steroid-sparing drugs such as methotrexate and azathioprine
- Mortality is most commonly a result of pulmonary and cardiac complications.

Physiology Correlation. Patients with DM and interstitial lung disease present with dyspnea on exertion. A restrictive pattern on pulmonary function tests is typical and is characterized by reduced total lung capacity (TLC) <80% of the predicted value. This can lead to pulmonary hypertension and eventually to cor pulmonale, a form of right heart failure.

Pharmacology Correlation. High-dose prednisone is the first-line treatment for DM. Steroids are tapered down to the lowest effective dose over 1 year, and patients are maintained on low-dose steroid therapy for 1–3 years. Systemic steroids have serious complications including osteoporosis and vertebral body compression fractures, weight gain, hypertension, diabetes, and lipid abnormalities. Avascular necrosis (AVN) is another common steroid-related complication and should be considered in any patient on steroids with new joint-related pain.

Musculoskeletal

Vignette 7

A 60-year-old man arrives at the ED with an acute onset left distal thigh pain. He has had a deep, dull, achy pain at this same site for the past year. The acute pain started after minimal trauma while stumbling off a curb. There is no other acute trauma. Left knee x-rays show a 7 cm intramedullary lucent lesion in the distal femur with irregular "rings-and-arcs" type matrix mineralization. The bone cortex adjacent to the lesion is destroyed and there is aggressive-appearing periosteal reaction.

Pathogenesis. Chondrosarcoma is a malignant tumor of cartilage and the second most common primary bone sarcoma after osteosarcoma. It is the most common bone sarcoma in adults. Chondrosarcoma can occur de novo or can arise from malignant degeneration of common benign cartilage tumors such as enchondromas or osteochondromas.

Clinical Presentation. Chondrosarcoma can present at any age but is more common in middle-aged adults. Men > women. The long bones and axial skeleton are common locations, and the tumors are typically large (>5 cm) at the time of diagnosis. Localized chronic, deep pain at the site of the tumor is typical. Pain is often worse at night. If there is cortical destruction and an associated soft tissue component of the tumor, a firm palpable mass may be present. Patients can present with acute onset of pain and disability if there is a pathologic fracture. Neurologic and vascular symptoms occur when the tumor invades or displaces adjacent nerves and blood vessels. The lungs and other bones are the most common sites of chondrosarcoma metastases.

Diagnostic Studies.

- Plain x-rays (initial diagnostic test), obtained prior to MRI; x-rays can show tumor-associated cortical destruction, aggressive periosteal reaction, and pathologic fractures
  - Radiographic pattern of mineralization in cartilage tumors has "rings-and-arcs" configuration
  - This pattern differs from the "cloud-like" mineralization pattern seen with osteoblastic tumors like osteosarcoma
- CT and MRI to delineate local extent of the tumor, including any soft tissue component
- Chest CT to evaluate for pulmonary metastases

Morphologic Features.

- Gross examination: white to blue tumor in medullary cavity eroding or thickening adjacent cortex; myxoid change
- Microscopy: sheets of cartilage-producing cells
  - Most common histologic subtype is "conventional" chondrosarcoma
  - Grading is based on cellularity and nuclear atypia of the chondrocytes

Differential Diagnosis. Differentiating high-grade chondrosarcoma from other primary malignant bone sarcomas is typically based on clinical history and radiographic appearance. Osteosarcoma and Ewing sarcoma (the first and third most common primary bone sarcomas, respectively) occur in a younger age group. Mineralization in bone forming tumors such as osteosarcoma has a fluffy or "cloud-like" configuration rather than the "rings-and-arcs" pattern of matrix mineralization seen with cartilage tumors like chondrosarcoma. In patients age >50, metastases to bone from other tumors are more common than primary bone sarcomas. The radiographic appearance of the sclerotic bone metastases of breast and prostate cancer, in particular, can mimic a primary cartilaginous bone tumor. History of known malignancy is the key factor.

Treatment and Outcomes.

- Surgery (primary treatment)
- Chondrosarcoma is typically resistant to both radiation and chemotherapy.
- Histologic grading is one of the most important prognostic factors with cartilage tumors. Chondrosarcoma is graded into 3 groups based on nuclear size, degree of cellularity, mitotic activity and staining pattern.
  - Grade 1 (low-grade) chondrosarcoma: <1% chance of metastases
  - Grade 3 chondrosarcoma: up to 70% of cases are metastatic

Physiology Correlation. Chemotherapy does not have an important role in the management of traditional intramedullary chondrosarcoma. That is because chemotherapy is typically useful for tumors that grow quickly, and chondrosarcoma grows slowly.

Pharmacology Correlation. Chemotherapy and radiation therapy may be effective in treating the mesenchymal subtype of chondrosarcoma. This subtype is rare and has a worse prognosis compared to intramedullary chondrosarcoma. Adjuvant chemotherapy is chemotherapy administered after resection; neoadjuvant chemotherapy is administered prior to resection in cases where the tumor involves adjacent key anatomic structures that will complicate the resection of tumor.

Vignette 8

A 37-year-old man presents with lower back pain. He complains of stiffness in his axial spine that usually improves over the course of the morning with activity. X-ray of the lumbar spine is normal, while x-ray of the sacroiliac joints shows bilateral abnormality including irregular joint space widening with bone erosions and subchondral sclerosis. HLA-B27 is positive.

Pathogenesis. Ankylosing spondylitis (AS) is the prototypical seronegative spondyloarthropathy. The seronegative spondyloarthropathies include ankylosing spondylitis, spondyloarthropathy associated with inflammatory bowel disease (IBD), psoriatic arthritis, and reactive arthritis. AS is an inflammatory arthritis of the axial skeleton involving mainly the spine and sacroiliac joints. The second main site of inflammation in AS is at the attachment sites of tendons or ligaments to bone (entheses). This is referred to as enthesitis. In the spine and sacroiliac joints, chronic inflammation can result in eventual ossification and fusion of the joints referred to as ankylosis.

Clinical Presentation. AS is common in males, with disease onset age <40. Inflammatory-type back pain (worse in the morning, improved by exercise and not relieved by rest) and stiffness are typical presenting symptoms. Later in the disease process, rigidity in the spine from bony ankylosis predisposes to spinal fracture after minor trauma. Pain at tendon or ligamentous insertions represents the enthesitis associated with AS. This commonly occurs at the heel, involving the Achilles tendon and plantar fascia. Extraskeletal manifestations of AS are commonly seen in the eyes, heart, lungs and bowel.

Diagnostic Studies.
- Genetic testing for HLA-B27 (strong association with AS)
- Rheumatoid factor and ANAs negative
- Spine radiographs show syndesmophytes and the so-called "shiny corner" sign in early disease and spinal fusion in late disease including the development of the bamboo spine with ankylosis
- Sacroiliac joint radiographs show sacroiliitis with sacroiliac joint space widening, subchondral sclerosis and bone erosions
- MRI of the spine and sacroiliac joints is the only imaging modality that can show active inflammation (bone marrow edema) in the spine or sacroiliac joints

Musculoskeletal

Morphologic Features.
- Sacroiliac joint is composed of 2 distinct portions
  - Anterior inferior segment of the joint is a true synovial joint lined by hyaline cartilage
  - Posterior superior portion is a fibrocartilaginous union
- Synovial portion of the joint is involved by a joint-centered inflammatory arthritis; the posterior-superior segment demonstrates the manifestations of AS-associated enthesopathy

Differential Diagnosis. AS can be distinguished from the other seronegative spondyloarthropathies by clinical history and disease distribution. Psoriatic arthritis and reactive arthritis more commonly involve the appendicular skeleton (hand and feet) and the sacroiliac joint disease is more commonly unilateral rather than bilateral and symmetric as is seen with AS. Look for characteristic skin lesions with psoriatic arthritis and the typical history of arthritis, uveitis and urethritis or cervicitis with reactive arthritis. Osteoarthritis is a very common cause of back pain and can be distinguished from AS by the absence of inflammatory-type back pain. The back pain in osteoarthritis is made worse, not better, with activity or exercise.

Treatment and Outcomes.
- Physical therapy and NSAIDs (first-line treatment)
- Tumor necrosis factor (TNF) inhibitors for NSAID-refractory disease
- Surgical intervention for fracture stabilization

Physiology Correlation. Cardiac manifestations of AS are seen in up to 10% of patients and include aortitis, aortic valve insufficiency and pericarditis. Aortic regurgitation is common and is described as a high-pitched decrescendo murmur of early diastole. This murmur is heard best at the third intercostal space on the left (Erb's point) with the patient sitting up and leaning forward.

Pharmacology Correlation. TNF inhibitors are used in AS patients with active inflammation refractory to NSAID therapy. This class of medications is most effective in preventing disease progression when initiated in the early stages of the illness, prior to the development of structural changes in the joint. This practice has increased the use of MRI in the diagnosis and management of AS patients because MRI is the only modality that can show inflammation prior to the development of irreversible joint destruction.

Vignette 9

An 18-year-old man presents with a painless, enlarging right thigh soft tissue mass for 3 months. He reports no history of prior thigh trauma. Physical exam reveals a hard, nonmobile and noncompressible soft tissue mass. Plain x-ray shows a noncalcified soft tissue mass measuring 10 cm.

Pathogenesis. Rhabdomyosarcoma is the most common childhood soft tissue sarcoma and is one of the round blue cell tumors of childhood, which include Ewing sarcoma, lymphoma and neuroblastoma. It is a malignant tumor of muscle origin. Most rhabdomyosarcomas are isolated tumors. Familial syndromes associated with increased risk of rhabdomyosarcoma include neurofibromatosis type-1, Li-Fraumeni syndrome (p53 tumor suppressor protein mutation), and Beckwith-Wiedemann syndrome.

Clinical Presentation. Extremity sarcomas typically present as a painless enlarging soft tissue mass as in vignette 9. Additional signs and symptoms depend on the specific tumor location. Orbital tumors present with proptosis or visual disturbances; prostate tumors can present with bowel or bladder dysfunction; uterine or urinary bladder masses may present with menorrhagia or hematuria.

- Embryonal subtype is most common in young children (age <5 years); it is seen most often in the head/neck, genital region, and urinary tract.
- Alveolar subtype is most common in older children and teenagers; it is seen most often in the muscles of the trunk and extremities.

Diagnostic Studies.

- Plain radiographs of soft tissue masses are nonspecific but required prior to MRI.
- MRI provides superior characterization of soft tissue masses and guides biopsy.
- Percutaneous image guided biopsy or surgical biopsy required for definitive diagnosis.

Morphologic Features.

- Gross examination: tumors growing into body cavities are polypoid with a glistening cut surface and foci of hemorrhage or cyst formation; intramuscular tumors are infiltrative with a bulging cut surface.
- Microscopic examination: sheets of poorly differentiated, round, blue cells with an eccentrically placed nucleus. Areas of hypercellularity alternate with sparsely cellular myxoid areas. Cross striations are not present in every case.

Differential Diagnosis. A palpable mass may be a benign or malignant soft tissue tumor or may be nonneoplastic such as a hematoma or abscess. Most pediatric soft tissue tumors are benign, with hemangioma being the most common benign tumor. Clinical history is critical when determining the need for additional workup of a mass. Any soft tissue mass that is rapidly enlarging or painful requires further evaluation. Immunohistochemistry staining for muscle-related proteins including actin, myosin, desmin, and myoglobin will help distinguish rhabdomyosarcoma from other small round blue cell tumors.

Treatment and Outcomes.

- Surgery, chemotherapy, and radiation all play an important role in treatment.
- Patient age and tumor characteristics are important prognostic factors.

Physiology Correlation. Muscle fibers show microscopic transverse striations. There are dark and light bands in striated muscle. The Z-line runs through the center of the light band. The sarcomere is the contractile unit of the muscle. During muscle contraction, the sarcomere shortens and the Z-lines move closer together.

Pharmacology Correlation. The VAC regimen that is used to treat rhabdomyosarcoma is vincristine, dactinomycin (actinomycin-D), and cyclophosphamide. An adverse effect of vincristine is a dose-related peripheral neurotoxicity. Most chemotherapy-induced neuropathies are sensory. The symptoms include sensory loss (e.g., problems with gait) and positive sensory perceptions (e.g., paresthesia).

Musculoskeletal

Vignette 10

> A 21-year-old man arrives at the ED from a construction site. His right lower extremity was trapped under a metal beam for 1 hour prior to extrication. There is evidence of blunt trauma to the right thigh, but there is no obvious penetrating injury. Lab evaluation reveals hyperkalemia and severe elevation of creatine kinase (CK).

Pathogenesis. Rhabdomyolysis is a severe muscle injury most commonly associated with prolonged immobilization from alcohol or drug abuse, trauma, or exposure to certain medications. Muscle breakdown releases massive amounts of potentially toxic intracellular contents into the blood. Released muscle elements can damage the kidneys resulting in acute renal failure. Hyperkalemia results from release of potassium from damaged muscle and can lead to life-threatening arrhythmia.

Clinical Presentation. The classic triad of rhabdomyolysis is muscle pain, muscle weakness, and dark urine. Other presenting symptoms depend on the precipitating mechanism (trauma, infection, medications).

Diagnostic Studies.
- Serum CK levels typically 10× the upper limit of normal
- Serum chemistry analysis to evaluate for critical electrolyte disturbances and renal dysfunction
- Urine dipstick positive for blood with few or no RBCs is suggestive of myoglobinuria
- Measure muscle compartment pressures if concern for compartment syndrome

Morphologic Features.
- The diagnosis is based on clinical findings (not morphology). At fasciotomy, operative findings can include hematoma (compressing adjacent nerves and vessels) and gangrene.
- Microscopic findings in necrotic muscle: **Coagulative necrosis** preserves cell outlines; liquefactive necrosis is seen later in the course.

Differential Diagnosis. Inflammatory myopathies can present with symptoms of muscle pain and weakness along with elevated CK levels. The chronicity of symptoms helps differentiate them from rhabdomyolysis, and muscle biopsy confirms the diagnosis of inflammatory myopathy. Myalgia from other common etiologies such as viral infection (influenza) or fibromyalgia can be distinguished by the clinical history and are not associated with a significant rise in CK levels.

Treatment and Outcomes.

- Immediate and aggressive IV fluid hydration (critical for preventing renal injury)
- Correction of electrolyte abnormalities (for preventing life-threatening arrhythmia)
- Relief of compartment syndrome with fasciotomy when necessary

Physiology Correlation. Rhabdomyolysis can be associated with compartment syndrome after acute extremity injury. Compartment syndrome results when the pressure in a muscle compartment due to swelling exceeds the perfusion pressure. Increased compartment pressures can lead to neurovascular compromise of the involved extremity. Compartment pressures >30 mm Hg (normal <15 mm Hg) require surgical evaluation for possible fasciotomy.

Pharmacology Correlation. Mannitol and sodium bicarbonate can be used in conjunction with aggressive hydration in the treatment of rhabdomyolysis. Alkalization of urine with bicarbonate decreases the acute tubular necrosis (ATN) that occurs in the context of acidic urine. Mannitol is an osmotic diuretic that increases urinary output and decreases renal tubular obstruction from the myoglobin casts.

Musculoskeletal

Test What You Have Learned

1. A 52-year-old woman is evaluated for weakness in her legs. Strength testing is notable for weakness of her proximal leg muscles, and to lesser degree her proximal arm muscles. Her hands show Gottron papules and her face has periorbital edema with a purplish hue. Which of the following problems related to her disease would she be most likely to have?

    A. Acute monoarticular arthritis

    B. Blindness

    C. Cranial nerve compression

    D. Genu varum

    E. Interstitial lung disease

    F. Podagra

2. A 44-year-old woman consults a physician because she has noticed that the upper part of her right arm is now wider than her left. She describes having had increasing pain in the right arm for several years which she attributed to muscle soreness. Physical examination demonstrates that her right humerus has increased diameter over the upper one-third of the shaft. Which of the following findings on further studies would most likely establish the probable diagnosis?

    A. Altered muscle contractility on electromyographic testing

    B. Cortical and medullary thickening of the bone

    C. Crystals on shoulder joint aspiration

    D. Cupping, fraying, and splaying of metaphyses

    E. Decreased bone density

    F. "Rings and arcs" mineralization

3. A 3-year-old girl is taken to the ED due to a possible broken arm. X-rays show a recent fracture of the radius and several older fractures elsewhere in her body. Weeks later, child abuse is ruled out and a thorough evaluation reveals a genetic disease. Although a bone biopsy was not performed, what microscopic features would be expected in this case?

    A. Aggressive osteoblastic activity with increased woven bone formation

    B. Muscle fiber necrosis

    C. Needle-shaped and negatively birefringent crystals

    D. Positive immunostaining for myoglobin

    E. Rhomboid shaped and positively birefringent crystals

    F. Thickened and ill-defined growth plate

    G. Thin cortex with rudimentary trabeculae

4. A 12-month-old girl is brought to a physician because she cries every time she tries to walk. Her mother has been almost exclusively breastfeeding her daughter because she was told that breast milk helps the baby's immune system. The mother and daughter reside in Alaska. Which of the following laboratory results would establish the likely diagnosis?

   A. Elevated serum creatine kinase

   B. High serum phosphorus

   C. Low urinary calcium

   D. Synovial fluid WBC >50,000/mcL

   E. Synovial fluid with needle-shaped crystals

   F. Urine positive for blood on dipstick with no red blood cells microscopically

5. A 65-year-old woman consults a physician because the skin on her face feels too tight to her. The patient has also been experiencing tingling sensations on her face. Physical examination demonstrates that the patient's facial bones are enlarged, particularly the mandible. Which of the following medications would be most helpful to her?

   A. Bicarbonate to alkalinize urine

   B. Biphosphonates

   C. Colchicine

   D. Doxycycline

   E. Mannitol

   F. TNF inhibitors

Answers: 1. (E), 2. (F), 3. (G), 4 (C), 5. (B)

CHAPTER 4
Endocrine System

Developmental Disorders

- ❏ Congenital hypopituitarism
- ❏ Persistent thyroglossal duct
- ❏ Congenital hypothyroidism
- ❏ Congenital absence of parathyroid
- ❏ Congenital absence of adrenal
- ❏ Congenital adrenal hyperplasia
- ❏ Heterotopic pancreas
- ❏ Annular pancreas

Autoimmune Disease

- ❏ Hashimoto thyroiditis
- ❏ Graves disease
- ❏ Addison disease
- ❏ Autoimmune polyendocrinopathy-candidiasis-ectodermal dystrophy

Trauma

- ❏ Endocrine disorders following traumatic brain injury

Inflammatory Disease

- ❏ Subacute thyroiditis

Infectious Disease

- ❏ Endocrine complications of HIV

System-Specific Processes

- ❏ Diabetes mellitus
- ❏ Gestational diabetes
- ❏ Hyperpituitarism and hypopituitarism
- ❏ Hyperthyroidism and hypothyroidism
- ❏ Goiter
- ❏ Hyperparathyroidism and hypoparathyroidism
- ❏ Hyperadrenalism and adrenal insufficiency

Neoplasias

- ❏ Pituitary adenomas
- ❏ Thyroid carcinoma: papillary, follicular, anaplastic, medullary
- ❏ Follicular adenoma
- ❏ Parathyroid adenoma
- ❏ Adrenal adenoma
- ❏ Endocrine tumors of the pancreas
- ❏ Multiple endocrine neoplasia: type 1, 2A and 2B

Representative Diseases

What follows are clinical vignettes for 10 select diseases within this organ system. First, read the vignette and try to identify the condition. Then, move on to read integrated information on each disease.

Vignette 1

A 52-year-old man with AIDS presents to the ED with lightheadedness, fatigue, and nausea. He also complains of chronic diarrhea, weight loss, and difficulty swallowing. On examination his pulse is 98/min, blood pressure 80/50 mm Hg, and temperature 38.6 C (101.5 F). Sodium level is low.

Diagnosis? _____

Vignette 2

A 46-year-old man with small cell lung cancer is brought to the ED by a friend, who states that the cancer patient is suffering from new onset of confusion. Laboratory evaluation reveals serum sodium 120 mmol/L and urine osmolality in excess of plasma osmolality. According to electronic medical records, last month the patient's serum sodium was WNL.

Diagnosis? _____

Vignette 3

During a postpartum checkup, a 29-year-old woman complains that she has been feeling unwell and also wonders why she has not been able to breastfeed her infant (lactation failure). The birth history is significant for placenta previa.

Diagnosis? _____

Vignette 4

A 42-year-old man complains to his physician that he has trouble concentrating at work. He also has symptoms of carpal tunnel syndrome and has gained weight. On physical examination the thyroid gland is diffusely enlarged.

Diagnosis? _____

Vignette 5

A 51-year-old man is found to have a palpable thyroid nodule during his annual health screening. He reports he has been having diarrhea, which he attributes to stress at work. His primary care doctor refers him to a specialist for fine-needle aspiration (FNA).

Diagnosis? _____

Endocrine

Vignette 6

A 43-year-old woman comes to the clinic with months of extreme fatigue. She was hospitalized a month ago for pancreatitis and has since recovered, but she still continues to have some abdominal pain. She says she "aches all over" and does not feel like going out with her friends anymore. Subsequent workup shows hypercalcemia, high parathyroid hormone levels, and cystic bone changes on x-ray.

Diagnosis? _____

Vignette 7

A 56-year-old woman has trouble concentrating, sleeping, and socializing with others. She feels anxious and tired all the time. She also experiences numbness and tingling around her lips and hands.

Diagnosis? _____

Vignette 8

A 38-year-old man comes to the ED due to unremitting epigastric pain and bloody urine. Physical examination reveals costovertebral tenderness. Abdominal CT shows a kidney stone in the right ureter. CT also shows a mass in the duodenum. Subsequent lab tests show high calcium, high PTH, and high gastrin.

Diagnosis? _____

Vignette 9

A 43-year-old woman presents with a 5-month history of episodic headaches accompanied by sweating and heart palpitations. She reports that one day she had an episode in the grocery store. During the attack, she was able to take her blood pressure at the kiosk in the store, and it was elevated.

Diagnosis? _____

Endocrine

Vignette 10

A 50-year-old man with type 2 diabetes mellitus (DM) comes to the clinic because of persistent rash and blisters on his arm. He has lost 15 pounds over the past 3 months. Labs show increased glucagon and glucose.

Diagnosis? _____

Vignette 1

A 52-year-old man with AIDS presents to the ED with lightheadedness, fatigue, and nausea. He also complains of chronic diarrhea, weight loss, and difficulty swallowing. On examination his pulse is 98/min, blood pressure 80/50 mm Hg, and temperature 38.6 C (101.5 F). Sodium level is low.

Pathogenesis. Primary chronic adrenal insufficiency (Addison's disease) is a type of adrenocortical hypofunction. Causes of Addison's include autoimmune disease, cancer, and infection. Pathogens such as CMV can induce inflammatory fibrosis in the adrenal glands (especially the cortex), destroying the ability to produce aldosterone, glucocorticoids, and sex hormones. Metabolic derangements such as hyponatremia, hyperkalemia, and hypoglycemia ensue.

Clinical Presentation. The clinical presentation of chronic adrenal insufficiency is insidious and nonspecific. Symptoms include nausea, fatigue, weakness and hypotension. Hyponatremia is present in the majority of patients at presentation. Stress (surgery, trauma, etc.) in a patient with chronic adrenal insufficiency can cause acute adrenal crisis, which may present with vomiting, abdominal pain, and a rapid spiral to hypovolemic shock.

Diagnostic Studies.
- Cosyntropin stimulation test; cortisol levels will be low after stimulation with ACTH
- Plasma ACTH is high in primary adrenal insufficiency
- PCR (polymerase chain reaction) is preferred method for CMV diagnosis

Morphologic Features.
- Gross examination of adrenal glands: The pathologic changes vary with the etiology of the adrenal hypofunction. Autoimmune adrenalitis causes a reduction in the size of the glands.
- Microscopy: If an infectious etiology causes the hypofunction, granulomas may be seen if the pathogen is tuberculosis or fungus.

Differential Diagnosis. Another cause of severe hypotension with or without fever is septic shock (following the flu, pneumonia, urinary tract infection, etc.) especially in a vulnerable patient population like the elderly. In an inflammatory state, however, one would expect high, not low, levels of cortisol. Acute adrenal crisis may present with features of acute abdomen.

Treatment and Outcomes.

- Glucocorticoid (hydrocortisone) and mineralocorticoid (fludrocortisone) replacement therapy.
- Adrenal androgen replacement therapy is considered optional.

Physiology Correlation. Primary adrenal insufficiency causes hyperpigmentation due to ACTH stimulation of melanocytes; in secondary adrenal insufficiency, hyperpigmentation does not occur because ACTH is not elevated. In secondary adrenal insufficiency, aldosterone production is maintained so serum potassium is normal.

Pharmacology Correlation. Patients treated for other diseases with exogenous steroids may experience iatrogenic adrenal insufficiency because exogenous steroids inhibit the natural production of steroids in the adrenal glands.

Vignette 2

A 46-year-old man with small cell lung cancer is brought to the ED by a friend, who states that the cancer patient is suffering from new onset of confusion. Laboratory evaluation reveals serum sodium 120 mmol/L and urine osmolality in excess of plasma osmolality. According to electronic medical records, last month the patient's serum sodium was WNL.

Pathogenesis. Syndrome of inappropriate antidiuretic hormone (SIADH) is a problem with osmoregulation due to secretion of arginine vasopressin (AVP) that may be due to a number of causes including drugs, neurologic disease, infection and ectopic release of AVP from neoplasms. There is a rare genetic variant.

Clinical Presentation. Symptoms include nausea, vomiting, muscle cramps, and neuropsychiatric manifestations (personality changes, seizures, hallucinations and even coma).

Diagnostic Studies.
- Diagnosis of exclusion
- Euvolemic hyponatremia
- If family members are also affected, sequencing of the V2 receptor gene

Morphologic Features.
- The diagnosis of SIADH is based on clinical features and not morphology.
- Cerebral edema causes flattening of gyri.

Differential Diagnosis.
- Diuretic abuse
- Secondary adrenal insufficiency

Treatment and Outcomes.
- Most cases are self-limiting, but a minority of cases do not resolve and lapse into chronicity.
- The genetic variant is a permanent condition.
- Treatment of hyponatremia is corrected gradually and with laboratory monitoring; fluid restriction may be necessary.

Endocrine

Physiology Correlation. Expansion of intracellular volume from hyponatremia causes brain swelling and increases intracranial pressure.

Pharmacology Correlation. Drugs causing SIADH include vasopressin, serotonin reuptake inhibitors, oxytocin, vincristine, carbamazepine, nicotine, and phenothiazines.

Vignette 3

During a postpartum checkup, a 29-year-old woman complains that she has been feeling unwell and also wonders why she has not been able to breastfeed her infant (lactation failure). The birth history is significant for placenta previa.

Pathogenesis. Sheehan syndrome (SS) is a form of **hypopituitarism due to ischemic necrosis** secondary to postpartum hemorrhage and hypovolemia. It can affect production of TSH, LH, FSH, GH, ACTH and prolactin. Pituitary apoplexy is enlargement of the gland secondary to ischemia or necrosis; it is seen with SS but it is also associated with pituitary adenoma. SS is more common in developing countries with suboptimal obstetric care.

Clinical Presentation. Symptoms begin days or years after childbirth. The condition may present emergently with seizure or coma, although this presentation is rare. Patients may complain of headache or feeling unwell in general; alternatively, some patients have complaints attributable to pituitary hormone deficiency with its consequent hyponatremia and hypoglycemia. The most common symptoms are **failure to lactate** (vignette 3) **or failure to resume menstruation** in the months following childbirth.

Diagnostic Studies.

- Hyponatremia is the most common electrolyte abnormality at presentation.
- Laboratory measurement of effector organ hormone levels that are regulated by the pituitary, for example, T_4. Assays of basal levels and stimulation levels (dynamic testing) are obtained.
- MRI with contrast for imaging of the pituitary gland; pituitary enlargement (early) or empty sella (late).

Morphologic Features.

- Gross features: At autopsy for pituitary insufficiency, sometimes only a small amount of pituitary tissue remains visible in the sella turcica (empty sella).
- Microscopic examination of pituitary biopsy shows pale shadows of infarcted cells in early cases; fibrosis is seen in cases biopsied later in the course.

Differential Diagnosis. It is important to consider Sheehan syndrome in a postpartum patient presenting with signs of postpartum depression. Careful inquiry about birth history, lactation and resumption of menstruation may lead to a laboratory investigation of pituitary function.

Treatment and Outcomes.

- Long-standing hormonal deficiency necessitates lifelong hormone replacement therapy
- A complication of SS is adrenal crisis

Physiology Correlation. The anterior pituitary secretes trophic hormones. The basophils secrete hormones (TSH, ACTH, LH and FSH) that control the activities of endocrine effector organs. Prolactin and growth hormone (the acidophils) also act on target organs that are not endocrine.

Pharmacology Correlation. The anterior pituitary is important for the neuroendocrine response to stress. When patients are under stress due to illness, trauma or surgery, adjustments to the dosage of corticosteroids is necessary.

Vignette 4

A 42-year-old man complains to his physician that he has trouble concentrating at work. He also has symptoms of carpal tunnel syndrome and has gained weight. On physical examination the thyroid gland is diffusely enlarged.

Pathogenesis. Hashimoto thyroiditis (HT) is an autoimmune destruction of the thyroid glands by antithyroperoxidase antibodies and is one of the most common causes of hypothyroidism. Low levels of free T4 cause an appropriate increase in TSH from the anterior pituitary. The incidence of HT is increasing (~2% of the U.S. population) and may be due to increased dietary iodine.

Clinical Presentation. A goiter may or may not be present. Patients may be asymptomatic or may have symptoms of hypothyroidism. In early stages, there may be cold intolerance, brittle hair, dry skin, myalgia, fatigue, depression, and weight gain. Carpal tunnel syndrome may also occur. In later stages, there may be hoarseness, myxedema, and atherosclerosis.

Diagnostic Studies.
- Thyroid hormone levels vary:
  - Hypothyroid: low thyroid hormone levels (free T4) with elevated TSH
  - Euthyroid
  - Subclinically hypothyroid: normal thyroid levels with elevated TSH
- Thyroid U/S: enlargement with hypoechoic micronodules
- Elevated serum thyroid peroxidase antibody and thyroglobulin antibody

Morphologic Features.
- Gross examination of the thyroid: symmetric glandular enlargement
- Microscopy: eosinophilic change of follicular epithelium and lympho-cytic infiltrate forming germinal centers

Differential Diagnosis. In rare cases when the gland is tender, subacute thyroiditis may be a diagnostic consideration. Hyperthyroidism may also cause goiter. The radioactive iodine uptake test is a diagnostic tool that is complementary to thyroid hormone levels in distinguishing between these entities.

Treatment and Outcomes.
- Lifelong replacement therapy with levothyroxine in some cases
- The clinical course is variable and requires monitoring of TSH levels
- B-cell thyroid lymphoma is a rare complication

Endocrine

Physiology Correlation. Thyroid hormones are involved in collagen synthesis and TSH receptors can be found on fibroblasts. Myxedema in hypothyroidism is a thickening of the skin (nonpitting) that occurs due to a build-up of glycosaminoglycans (GAG) made by the fibroblasts. Hypothyroidism increases capillary permeability, leading to an increase of albumin and other proteins in the interstitium.

Pharmacology Correlation. Levothyroxine is a very common medication that easily replaces thyroid hormones in patients with hypothyroidism. Patients with celiac disease or inflammatory bowel disease are predisposed to a decreased GI absorption of levothyroxine, and the dosage may need to be increased. Women are usually also treated with an increased dose during pregnancy.

Vignette 5

A 51-year-old man is found to have a palpable thyroid nodule during his annual health screening. He reports he has been having diarrhea, which he attributes to stress at work. His primary care doctor refers him to a specialist for fine-needle aspiration (FNA).

Pathogenesis. Medullary thyroid carcinoma (MTC) is a neuroendocrine tumor arising from the parafollicular C cells of the thyroid. The majority of cases arise spontaneously, but a quarter of cases are familial. The hereditary forms often have C cell hyperplasia in the parenchyma surrounding the tumor; this lesion may be a tumor precursor. Thyroid cancers are uncommon and nonepithelial thyroid carcinoma is quite rare. MTC accounts for 5% of all thyroid cancers, but its association with MEN-2A (MTC, hyperparathyroidism and pheochromocytoma) makes it an important diagnostic entity.

Clinical Presentation. The most common presentation of MTC is an asymptomatic solitary thyroid nodule. When the nodule is palpable, the risk of spread to lymph nodes is higher. Diarrhea (vignette 5) is a rare presenting sign caused by tumor secretion of calcitonin and/or VIP.

Diagnostic Studies.

- Fine needle aspiration (FNA) is often a first step in the evaluation of thyroid nodules.
- Calcitonin is a tumor biomarker with high sensitivity for MTC.
- Neck U/S allows assessment of size, identification of other nodules, and status of lymph node involvement.
- *RET* molecular analysis is used for prognosis, treatment, and genetic counseling.
- Carcinoembryonic antigen (CEA) can be used to follow patients postoperatively.

Morphologic Features.

- Cytologic features of the FNA: hypercellularity, dispersed cells with a plasmacytoid appearance, neuroendocrine chromatin pattern, positive staining for calcitonin, amyloid identification with Congo-red staining
- Gross examination of the resected thyroid: tumor may be bilateral and multifocal
  - Some tumors are infiltrative
  - Cut surface may be soft or firm

- Microscopic examination of resected tumor: tumors vary in histologic appearance
    - Tumor cells may be round to spindled
    - The finding of amyloid in the stroma is a characteristic feature

Differential Diagnosis. Thyroid nodules are common (up to 50% of the U.S. adult population has one thyroid nodule). Most thyroid nodules are seen on imaging taken for other reasons. Size is a strong predictor of malignancy. The majority of cancerous nodules in the thyroid are papillary carcinoma, which has classic nuclear features (ground glass nuclei and nuclear grooves) and carries a good prognosis. The microscopic differential diagnosis of MTC includes metastatic neuroendocrine carcinoma, lymphoma and Hürtle cell carcinoma; measurement of serum calcitonin levels can be helpful.

Treatment and Outcomes.

- Total thyroidectomy with lymph node dissection of the central compartment.
- Radiotherapy has limited utility and is used in some cases for local control after surgery.
- Lymph node metastases occur in half of all cases; distant metastases occur in a fifth of cases.
- 10-year survival rate is >95% in cases confined to the thyroid.
- Levothyroxine replacement therapy

Physiology Correlation. Calcitonin is a calcium-lowering polypeptide hormone secreted by the C cells in the thyroid. Calcitonin level is sometimes ordered to screen individuals whose relatives have been diagnosed with MTC. Calcitonin level is also increased in renal insufficiency, hypercalcemia, and as a side effect of some drugs.

Pharmacology Correlation. Chronic use of omeprazole induces gastrin hypersecretion, and calcitonin secretion and synthesis are stimulated by high levels of gastrin. Beta-blockers also cause hypercalcitoninemia.

Endocrine

Vignette 6

A 43-year-old woman comes to the clinic with months of extreme fatigue. She was hospitalized a month ago for pancreatitis and has since recovered, but she still continues to have some abdominal pain. She says she "aches all over" and does not feel like going out with her friends anymore. Subsequent workup shows hypercalcemia, high parathyroid hormone levels, and cystic bone changes on x-ray.

Pathogenesis. Causes of **primary hyperparathyroidism** include parathyroid adenoma, diffuse or nodular hyperplasia, and carcinoma. Cases may occur sporadically or in association with MEN-1 or MEN-2A.

Clinical Presentation. Most patients are women age >50. An incidental finding of increased calcium during a laboratory investigation for other reasons is the common diagnostic watershed moment. The classic "bones, groans, stones, and moans" may not be present; patients may be asymptomatic or mildly symptomatic. Most of the hyperparathyroid symptoms arise from hypercalcemia. Hypercalcemia can cause pancreatitis as seen in the vignette. Other symptoms include fatigue, depression, and altered mental status.

Diagnostic Studies.
- High calcium (if primary hyperparathyroidism)
- High PTH
- High urine calcium
- X-ray shows cystic bone changes (also known as "salt and pepper" lesions)

Morphologic Features.
- Gross examination of parathyroid adenoma: solitary encapsulated mass compressing gland
- Microscopic examination of parathyroid adenoma: encapsulated lesion with sheets of chief cells

Differential Diagnosis. It is important to distinguish primary from secondary hyperparathyroidism. Both have symptoms of hypercalcemia, but secondary hyperparathyroidism has other symptoms associated with the root cause, e.g., chronic kidney disease.

Endocrine

Treatment and Outcomes.
- Surgery is 95% effective
- Bisphosphonates
- Cinacalcet
- Calcium and vitamin D
- Complications include hypertension, bone fracture, and kidney stones

Physiology Correlation. Neuronal and hormonal pathways affect gastric acid secretion. There are calcium-sensing receptors in the stomach. High calcium levels can increase gastrin production, causing gastric or duodenal ulcer.

Pharmacology Correlation. Furosemide functions by inhibiting the NaK2Cl cotransporter in the loop of Henle, thereby decreasing sodium, potassium, and chloride reabsorption. Normally, the reabsorbed potassium is recycled back out via Na^+/K^+ ATPase, which then generates an electrochemical gradient to passively reabsorb the magnesium and calcium, as potassium gets back out into the loop of Henle. However, when this gradient gets disrupted by furosemide, calcium no longer gets reabsorbed and excreted out, reducing calcium levels. Furosemide is still used as a treatment for hypercalcemia, but it is no longer considered one of the mainstays of treatment, as there are other more effective measures to decrease calcium levels.

Vignette 7

A 56-year-old woman has trouble concentrating, sleeping, and socializing with others. She feels anxious and tired all the time. She also experiences numbness and tingling around her lips and hands.

Pathogenesis. Idiopathic hypoparathyroidism is a term reserved for hypofunction of the parathyroids without a specific cause. Low parathyroid (PTH) levels cause low calcium, leading to neuromuscular dysfunction, calcification of the basal ganglia, and potentially fatal cardiac malfunction.

Clinical Presentation. Idiopathic hypoparathyroidism presents with symptoms of hypocalcemia. The early symptoms are neuromuscular and include muscle cramping and circumoral paresthesia. Later in the course, laryngospasm, bronchospasm and heart failure may occur.

Diagnostic Studies.
- Physical examination: **Chvostek sign** (twitching of facial muscles upon tapping of facial nerve over the parotid gland) and **Trousseau sign** (carpopedal spasm after inflation of BP cuff above systolic pressure).
- Laboratory investigation: parathyroid hormone, phosphate, magnesium, 25-hydroxyvitamin D, and corrected total calcium level
- Prolonged QT interval on EKG

Morphologic Features. Diagnosis is based on clinical information and not morphology.

Differential Diagnosis. The symptoms of tetany, seizures, and paresthesia lead to consideration of neurologic disorders. Other important causes of hypocalcemia include vitamin D deficiency and chronic renal failure. A clinical history is important because the most common cause of hypoparathyroidism is iatrogenic; the glands may be unintentionally destroyed or removed in patients undergoing thyroidectomy.

Treatment and Outcomes.
- Calcium and vitamin D replacement
- Mg replacement if needed
- Aluminum hydroxide (phosphate binders) to control hyperphosphatemia

Endocrine

Physiology Correlation. When calcium levels fall, PTH increases bone resorption to mobilize calcium, increases calcium absorption in the gastrointestinal tract, and increases reabsorption of calcium in the distal nephron.

Pharmacology Correlation. Albumin is the carrier protein for calcium. Because low albumin states (e.g., cirrhosis) impact the measurement of calcium, it is important to calculate a corrected calcium if the serum albumin is low. For every 1.0 g/dL drop in albumin, 0.8 must be added to the measured calcium to get the correct value.

Vignette 8

A 38-year-old man comes to the ED due to unremitting epigastric pain and bloody urine. Physical examination reveals costovertebral tenderness. Abdominal CT shows a kidney stone in the right ureter. CT also shows a mass in the duodenum. Subsequent lab tests show high calcium, high PTH, and high gastrin.

Pathogenesis. Multiple endocrine neoplasia-1 (MEN-1) is a rare autosomal dominant syndrome that affects the parathyroid (hyperplasia and adenoma), pancreas (lethal functioning tumors), and pituitary (prolactin macroadenoma). The syndrome is caused by mutation of the gene *MEN1*, which encodes the nuclear tumor suppressor protein, menin. Loss of functional menin allows unchecked cell division.

Clinical Presentation. Biochemical evidence of neoplasia may be present a decade before disease presents. Primary hyperparathyroidism usually presents first. One sign of hypercalcemia is formation of kidney stones, as seen in vignette 8. The phenotype is variable, and many other signs and symptoms are associated with the syndrome; for example, acromegaly may occur in the setting of a tumor that secretes somatotropin. Some important clinical features of multiple endocrine syndromes include: neoplasia occurring at a young age, multifocal tumors, and recurrent neoplasia.

Diagnostic Studies.
- Laboratory investigation of endocrine function
- Genetic testing for the mutation
- Screening for the neoplasms: imaging (CT, MRI, U/S), biochemical tests

Morphologic Features.
- Parathyroid: adenomas and hyperplasia
- Pancreas: pancreatic neuroendocrine tumors (pNETs), islet cell dysplasia/hyperplasia/tumors
- Pituitary: macroadenoma

Differential Diagnosis. The issue is often whether an endocrine tumor is sporadic or if it is associated with a multiple endocrine neoplasia syndrome. Inquiries about family history and testing for *MEN1* usually lead to a correct diagnosis, as long as a clinical suspicion for MEN exists.

Endocrine

Treatment and Outcomes.

- Genetic counseling and testing for family members
- Biochemical screening of affected individuals for early detection of neoplasia
- Early screening for breast cancer in females due to an increased incidence of breast cancer
- Surgical treatment as deemed necessary for the disease phenotype
- Size of pancreatic tumor correlates with metastases; malignant pNETs are the leading cause of death in MEN-1.
- Medical therapy to control endocrine hypersecretory states
- Chemotherapy and radiotherapy
- Increased risk of early death; MEN-1 has a 15-year survival that exceeds 90%.

Physiology Correlation. Zollinger-Ellison (ZE) syndrome is also known as gastrinoma, a tumor of gastrin-secreting cells in either the pancreas or duodenum. Gastrin stimulates parietal cells to increase HCl secretion, leading to peptic ulcer disease. Normally, secretin would decrease acid secretion; however, in the setting of gastrinoma, secretin fails to decrease gastrin levels. Persistently high gastrin levels after the secretin suppression test can confirm the diagnosis of ZE syndrome.

Pharmacology Correlation. Dopamine inhibits prolactin production in the anterior pituitary. The dopamine agonist cabergoline is useful in the treatment of prolactinoma.

Vignette 9

A 43-year-old woman presents with a 5-month history of episodic headaches accompanied by sweating and heart palpitations. She reports that one day she had an episode in the grocery store. During the attack, she was able to take her blood pressure at the kiosk in the store, and it was elevated.

Pathogenesis. Pheochromocytoma is a **catecholamine-secreting tumor** of the adrenal medulla or the sympathetic ganglia. These tumors cause hypertension when they secrete norepinephrine. The tumors may arise sporadically or may arise in association with **MEN-2A** (medullary thyroid carcinoma, pheochromocytoma, and hyperparathyroidism) and **MEN-2B** (medullary thyroid carcinoma, pheochromocytoma, marfanoid body habitus, and mucosal neuromas).

Clinical Presentation. The rule of 10s helps to remember features of clinical presentation: 10% are outside the adrenal, 10% are bilateral, 10% are found in children, 10% are not associated with hypertension.

The peak incidence is between the third and fifth decade of life. When the tumors secrete norepinephrine, they cause **sustained or episodic hypertension.** The classic presentation is paroxysmal attacks of hypertension accompanied by headache, perspiration and palpitation. Although some patients present in hypertensive crisis, others are normotensive. Some individuals with the tumor are asymptomatic, and their tumors come to medical attention only when an adrenal mass is an incidental imaging finding (incidental adrenaloma).

Diagnostic Studies.

- When CT or MRI shows an incidentaloma in adrenal gland, it must be determined if the tumor secretes catecholamines
- Lab assays to detect catecholamines and their metabolites, regardless of how a patient with pheochromocytoma presents
- **Plasma-fractionated metanephrines** or **24-hour urine metanephrines** (test of choice)

Morphologic Features.

- Gross examination: The tumors are more likely to be bilateral and multicentric in children. The encapsulated 3–5 cm tumors can appear to overtake the entire adrenal medulla. The cut surface is tan and occasionally hemorrhagic. The tumor may be solid or cystic.
- Microscopy: The tumor cells are arranged in cords and nests (Zellballen pattern). The nuclei are round and may be pleomorphic. The cytoplasm is granular and may contain PAS-positive hyaline globules.
- Electron microscopy: **Dense core granules** are seen. The granules contain a predominance of norepinephrine or epinephrine.

Differential Diagnosis. Headaches and hot flashes can also be present in hyperthyroidism. The headache pain is typically constant and not episodic; goiter and weight loss are usually also present.

Treatment and Outcomes.

- Surgical resection
- The presence of metastases (not nuclear pleomorphism) portends a worse prognosis.
- Most tumors are benign; 10% are malignant.

Physiology Correlation. Catecholamines are stored in electron-dense granules in the adrenal medulla; they are released in response to stress. Epinephrine has an effect on α and β receptors in blood vessels. Norepinephrine has a greater impact on α receptors. When α receptors are stimulated, vasoconstriction occurs; when β receptors are stimulated, vasodilatation occurs. Epinephrine and norepinephrine are metabolized to metanephrine and normetanephrine, respectively, and then the metanephrines are deaminated by MAO to vanillylmandelic acid (VMA). Catecholamines have a short half-life in the bloodstream, which is why measurement of urinary metabolites is ideal.

Pharmacology Correlation. Before surgery, patients with pheochromocytoma are treated with alpha blockers such as phenoxybenzamine in order to vasodilate and reduce BP. Alpha blockade must be achieved before beta blockade because if beta blockers get administered first, hypertensive crisis may ensue. When α adrenoreceptors are blocked first, sympathetic stimulation causes vasodilatation, not vasoconstriction.

Endocrine

Vignette 10

A 50-year-old man with type 2 diabetes mellitus (DM) comes to the clinic because of persistent rash and blisters on his arm. He has lost 15 pounds over the past 3 months. Labs show increased glucagon and glucose.

Pathogenesis. **Glucagonoma** is a tumor arising from the alpha cells of the pancreas, causing high levels of glucagon. Under normal circumstances, glucagon is released when serum glucose levels are low. Glucagonomas inappropriately release high levels of glucagon, stimulating gluconeogenesis and lipolysis to increase serum glucose levels.

Clinical Presentation. Glucagonoma has a very nonspecific presentation. It is frequently associated with DM due to hyperglycemia caused by the tumor, as shown in the vignette. Necrotizing migratory erythema causing irregular rashes and blisters on the extremities, shins, and buttocks is also associated with glucagonoma, but those are nonspecific findings since they are also associated with chronic pancreatitis, inflammatory bowel disease, and cirrhosis. This tumor also causes weight loss and fatigue.

Diagnostic Studies.
- High glucagon
- High glucose
- Low hemoglobin
- CT: mass in the pancreas

Morphologic Features.
- Tumor microscopy: gyriform pattern with glucagon + cells
- Necrotizing migratory erythema
  - Gross examination: erythematous papules with irregular borders; vesicles that crust
  - Microscopy: psoriasiform hyperplasia and perivascular lymphohistiocytic infiltrates

Differential Diagnosis. Because glucagonoma is a very rare tumor, it is worthwhile to consider MEN-1 syndrome as a differential in patients presenting with glucagonoma. While MEN-1 also involves the pancreas, MEN-1 patients may or may not have a family/personal history of cancer involving other MEN-1 organs (pituitary and parathyroid); testing for *MEN1* is helpful.

Endocrine

Treatment and Outcomes.

- Octreotide
- Surgical resection
- Metastasis worsens outcome

Physiology Correlation. High glucagon levels disrupt metabolic regulation by inappropriately activating both catabolic and anabolic pathways. There are subsequent deficiencies in fatty acids, amino acids, and important minerals such as zinc. These deficiencies will produce inflammation in the epidermis with even little trauma, which is the basis for necrotizing migratory erythema. It is also postulated that glucagon itself can cause these skin changes.

Pharmacology Correlation. Octreotide is a somatostatin analog which inhibits release of many products in the GI system, including but not limited to glucagon and insulin.

Test What You Have Learned

1. A 32-year-old woman is diagnosed with an endocrine tumor that secretes norepinephrine and causes symptoms of rapid onset of abdominal pain, palpitations, rapid breathing, dizziness, sweating, and headache. Which of the following laboratory findings was most helpful in establishing this patient's diagnosis?

   A. Anti-thyroperoxidase antibodies

   B. Early AM cortisol <5 ug/dL

   C. High calcitonin

   D. High glucacon

   E. High urine VMA

   F. Low corrected calcium

2. A 20-year-old man has a family history of endocrine disease. Following diagnosis of endocrine tumors in a relative, he underwent genetic testing, identifying *MEN1*. Elevation of which of the following would suggest pituitary involvement?

   A. ACTH

   B. Gastrin

   C. Glucagon

   D. Insulin

   E. PTH

   F. VIP

3. A 45-year-old woman consults a physician because she is having severe, persistent rashes and blisters on her extremities, shins, and buttocks. Laboratory studies demonstrate high glucose. CT scan of the abdomen shows a 3 cm mass of the pancreas. Which of the following medications would be most useful in therapy?

   A. Bisphonates

   B. Calcium

   C. IV steroids

   D. Levothyroxin

   E. Octreotide

   F. Tonivaptan

4. A woman presents with paroxysmal hypertension. Workup reveals a genetic mutation. Biopsy of the organ causing her symptoms would be most likely to show which of the following?

    A. Adenocarcinoma

    B. C-cell hyperplasia with amyloid deposits

    C. Monotonous cells with amyloid deposition

    D. Tumor cells with granular cytoplasm due to catecholamine-containing granules.

    E. Gyriform growth pattern

    F. Ground-glass nuclei

5. A 37-year-old woman undergoes thyroid biopsy of an enlarged thyroid gland. The biopsy shows marked loss of thyroid follicles with replacement by lymphoid tissue with germinal centers. This patient would be most likely to have which of the following?

    A. Altered mental status

    B. Hyperpituitarism

    C. Myxedema

    D. Necrotizing migratory erythema

    E. Thrombophlebitis

    F. Zollinger-Ellison syndrome

Answers: 1. (E), 2. (A), 3. (E), 4. (D), 5. (C)

CHAPTER 5

Cardiovascular System

Checklist of Processes Within This System

Developmental Disorders

- ❏ Congenital cardiac malformations
- ❏ Situs inversus
- ❏ Congenital hypertrophy

Trauma

- ❏ Hemopericardium
- ❏ Pericardial effusion

Infections

- ❏ Infective endocarditis

Inflammatory disease

- ❏ Myocarditis
- ❏ Rheumatic heart disease
- ❏ Endocarditis
- ❏ Pericarditis

System-Specific Processes

- ❏ Shock: cardiogenic, hypovolemic, septic
- ❏ Valvular disease: stenosis; prolapse
- ❏ Heart failure: right-sided; left-sided
- ❏ Conduction disturbances: afib; ventricular tachycardia; channelopathies
- ❏ Cardiomyopathy: dilated; hypertrophic; restrictive
- ❏ Diseases of the coronary arteries
- ❏ Myocardial infarction
- ❏ Cor pulmonale

Systemic disease affecting the heart

- ❏ Arteriosclerosis
  - ° Arteriolosclerosis
  - ° Monckeberg medial sclerosis
  - ° Fibromuscular intimal hyperplasia
  - ° Atherosclerosis
- ❏ Diseases of the great vessels
  - ° Aortic aneurysm/dissection
  - ° Marfan syndrome
- ❏ Hypertension
- ❏ Vasculitis of large, medium and small vessels
- ❏ Thrombotic disease
  - ° Nonbacterial thrombotic endocarditis
- ❏ Libman-Sacks endocarditis
- ❏ Drug reaction with eosinophilia and systemic symptoms (DRESS)
- ❏ Cardiac amyloidosis

Tumors

- ❏ Angiosarcoma
- ❏ Myxoma
- ❏ Rhabdomyoma

Representative Diseases

What follows are clinical vignettes for 10 select diseases within this organ system. First, read the vignette and try to identify the condition. Then, move on to read integrated information on each disease.

Vignette 1

After an uneventful pregnancy, an infant boy is born at 40 weeks gestation. A few hours after birth, the newborn nurse notices that the baby's nail beds are blue.

Diagnosis? _____

Vignette 2

A 39-year-old man with a history of IV drug use presents to the ED with sudden deafness in both ears. He is febrile.

Diagnosis? _____

Vignette 3

A 42-year-old woman, who states she was recently treated for a "skipping heart," comes to the ED in severe pain. She says the pain started about 24 hours ago after dinner. The pain is substernal and radiates through to her back; it worsens after eating. The patient says she also feels exhausted and nauseated. Electronic medical records reveal that she is taking amiodarone. Cardiac monitoring reveals regular rate and rhythm. Serum lipase is elevated.

Diagnosis? _____

Vignette 4

A 23-year-old woman is admitted to the hospital with rash, fever, and facial swelling. She states that 2 months ago she was treated for a UTI with trimethoprim/sulfamethoxazole. She is otherwise healthy. On her first night in the hospital, she experiences chest pain. An ECG shows ST-segment elevation, and cardiac necrosis biomarkers are significantly elevated.

Diagnosis? _____

Vignette 5

A 56-year-old-man with a 25 pack-year smoking history sees his physician with complaints of dyspnea and weight gain. Chest x-ray shows pulmonary artery enlargement and echo shows right ventricular hypertrophy.

Diagnosis? _____

Vignette 6

A woman brings her 70-year-old mother to the doctor, stating that she has been more fatigued and forgetful recently, and she has been complaining of difficulty breathing. Her mother has also had some "fainting spells."

Diagnosis? _____

Vignette 7

A 19-year-old-man sees his physician for a sports physical for basketball. He is slim and tall. Cardiac auscultation reveals a midsystolic murmur with click.

Diagnosis? _____

Vignette 8

A 64-year-old patient with chronic kidney disease comes to the ED complaining of pain "all over my chest." He had recently missed dialysis due to vacation. Auscultation reveals a friction rub. EKG is normal.

Diagnosis? _____

Vignette 9

A 3-year-old boy comes to the ED with spots on the abdomen. His mother reports he has had a fever for a week. Physical exam reveals conjunctivitis, mucositis, and edema of the hands and feet.

Diagnosis? _____

Vignette 10

A 3-month-old girl arrives at the ED with a seizure. Physical exam shows some light-brown patches on the left arm and a systolic murmur best heard in the apex.

Diagnosis? _____

Cardiovascular

Vignette 1

After an uneventful pregnancy, an infant boy is born at 40 weeks gestation. A few hours after birth, the newborn nurse notices that the baby's nail beds are blue.

Pathogenesis. **Transposition of the great arteries** (TGA) is a critical congenital heart defect that is a conotruncal (outflow) abnormality. It is one of the cardiac "5 T's" that causes cyanosis in newborns. The pulmonary artery arises from the left ventricle and the aorta arises from the right ventricle. This defect creates 2 parallel circuits of blood between the systemic and pulmonary circulations. About 9 in 1,000 live births have congenital heart disease. TGA is associated with maternal diabetes and is only rarely associated with extracardiac syndromes.

Clinical Presentation. Some cases of TGA are diagnosed prenatally with U/S screening. Others present with cyanosis and metabolic acidosis in the first hours after birth. Murmurs are typically not heard.

Diagnostic Studies.
- Prenatal fetal U/S screening (some cases can be missed)
- Pulse oximetry screening in the newborn nursery
- "Egg on a string" appearance on chest x-ray
- Echocardiography

Morphologic Features.
- D-transposition: aorta is to the right of pulmonary artery
- L-transposition: aorta is to the left of pulmonary artery

Differential Diagnosis.
Differential diagnosis for cyanotic heart defects in a newborn:
- Tetralogy of Fallot
- Transposition of the arteries
- Truncus arteriosus
- Tricuspid atresia
- Total anomalous pulmonary venous return

Cardiovascular

Treatment and Outcomes.

- Preoperatively, prostaglandin E1 to maintain patency of the ductus arteriosus
- Definitive surgical repair usually done in first week of life (almost always successful)

Physiology Correlation. The ductus arteriosus connects the aorta with the pulmonary artery, and it normally closes after birth. If it is allowed to remain open in an infant with TGA, it allows a mix of oxygen-rich and oxygen-poor blood.

Pharmacology Correlation. Prostaglandin E1 helps maintain patency of the ductus arteriosus to enable oxygenated blood from the pulmonary circulation to mix into the systemic circulation. It helps stabilize the infant prior to surgery.

Vignette 2

A 39-year-old man with a history of IV drug use presents to the ED with sudden deafness in both ears. He is febrile.

Pathogenesis. Acute endocarditis is infection with a high-virulence organism that damages cardiac valves. IV drug users are prone to acute endocarditis caused by *Staph aureus*. Valvular injury creates a nidus for platelet-fibrin formation and further infection, which leads to valvular vegetations.

Clinical Presentation. The most common presentation is fever. Other symptoms can arise, such as vascular hemorrhages (splinter hemorrhage, Janeway lesions), murmurs, and even hearing loss, as was the case in the vignette.

Diagnostic Studies.
- CBC, chem 7
- Blood cultures
- Echocardiogram
- Urinalysis

Morphologic Features.
- Valvular fibrinous vegetations
- Microscopically, vegetations are a collection of fibrin, platelets, bacteria, and lymphocytes with RBC debris

Differential Diagnosis. Bilateral sensorineural hearing loss is most commonly due to a systemic disease. Both endocarditis and rheumatic fever cause fever; however, acute endocarditis is an infection that occurs with a virulent organism and rheumatic fever is a type II hypersensitivity reaction from a previous Strep pharyngitis.

Treatment and Outcomes.
- IV antibiotic therapy
- Steroids are not used in cases with infectious etiology
- Cardiac valve surgery
- Cochlear implants; hearing loss is permanent

Cardiovascular

Physiology Correlation. Vegetations tend to occur where there is lower pressure of blood flow, which allows time for bacteria to infect and for platelet-fibrin complex to form.

Pharmacology Correlation. Empirically, when infectious endocarditis is suspected, broad-spectrum coverage of *Staph, Strep*, and *Enterococcus* is commenced (e.g., vancomycin and ceftriaxone). If cultures identify methicillin-sensitive *Staph aureus*, treatment with nafcillin or oxacillin is indicated.

Cardiovascular

Vignette 3

A 42-year-old woman, who states she was recently treated for a "skipping heart," comes to the ED in severe pain. She says the pain started about 24 hours ago after dinner. The pain is substernal and radiates through to her back; it worsens after eating. The patient says she also feels exhausted and nauseated. Electronic medical records reveal that she is taking amiodarone. Cardiac monitoring reveals regular rate and rhythm. Serum lipase is elevated.

Pathogenesis. Atrial fibrillation (AF) is the most common cause of clinical arrhythmia. Morphological and electrophysiological changes can cause disorganized atrial electrical activity. Ectopic beats can originate from the myocardial sleeve in pulmonary veins. Risk factors include advanced age, hypertension, cardiac surgery, mitral valve disease, cardiomyopathy, and thyrotoxicosis. Some cases are idiopathic.

Clinical Presentation. The ventricular rate in AF is 100–160 beats/minute. Some patients are asymptomatic, but when symptoms do occur they include palpitations, angina, and lightheadedness. Symptoms can be paroxysmal or persistent. When sinus rhythm cannot be maintained with medical therapy, the condition is called *permanent AF*. The patient in the vignette was being successfully managed with amiodarone but she developed acute pancreatitis as an adverse effect of therapy.

Diagnostic Studies.
- EKG to diagnose AF: irregularly irregular ventricular response (abnormal QRS complexes) with no P wave activity.
- Echocardiogram to assess underlying cardiac structural defects causing AF: valvular lesions or cardiac hypertrophy
- TSH/free T4 to rule out hyperthyroidism

Morphologic Features.
- Diagnosis of AF is based on clinical findings, but if a structural cardiac defect such as mitral valve pathology or cardiomyopathy underlies AF, changes related to that pathology will be present
- Changes in the atria due to AF include myocyte hypertrophy and fibroblast proliferation

Differential Diagnosis. Patients with palpitations are best evaluated with ECG while the symptoms are present. If patients are not symptomatic, hints from the medical history can be helpful. Patients with pulmonary disease may have atrial tachycardia. Listening to heart sounds is also helpful to uncover structural defects which can predispose to AF and ventricular tachycardia.

Cardiovascular

Lab investigation can help exclude anemia, hyperthyroidism and electrolyte abnormalities.

Treatment and Outcomes.
- Cardioversion (electrical or medical)
- Beta blockers, calcium channel blockers, and digoxin (to control ventricular rate)
- Sodium channel blockers and amiodarone (to restore sinus rhythm)
- Anticoagulants if needed (to prevent thromboembolic stroke)
- AV node ablation; radiofrequency ablation of pulmonary veins
- Complications of AF include heart failure, stroke and sudden death

Physiology Correlation. Patients with AF are at risk for thromboembolic events; hemostasis may cause thrombi to form in the atrium. Recall that Virchow's triad (hemodynamic changes, vessel injury or dysfunction, and hypercoagulability) explains the 3 main mechanisms for thrombosis.

Pharmacology Correlation. Amiodarone is one of many drugs (including statins, ACE inhibitors, and diuretics to name a few) that can cause acute pancreatitis. The mechanisms driving the adverse effect vary with the drugs. After ruling out other known causes of acute pancreatitis (gallstones, alcohol abuse, hyperlipidemia, and hypercalcemia), discontinuation of the drug in question leads to resolution of symptoms and correction of serum amylase and lipase.

Vignette 4

A 23-year-old woman is admitted to the hospital with rash, fever and facial swelling. She states that 2 months ago she was treated for a UTI with trimethoprim/sulfamethoxazole. She is otherwise healthy. On her first night in the hospital, she experiences chest pain. An ECG shows ST-segment elevation, and cardiac necrosis biomarkers are significantly elevated.

Pathogenesis. **Drug reaction with eosinophilia and systemic symptoms (DRESS)** is a T-cell mediated response to drug therapy that damages organs. It was previously known as drug rash with eosinophilia and systemic symptoms. The pathogenesis is not completely understood. The reaction may be mediated by an HLA-linked pharmacologic immune interaction. For example, HLA-B*5801 is associated with an allopurinol hypersensitivity reaction. It is theorized that the drug reaction alters the immune system and allows viral reactivation. There have been documented cases with associated HHV-6 reactivation. Other herpes viruses including EBV and CMV have also been implicated. Cases have been reported in children and adults.

Clinical Presentation. The **prolonged latent phase** of DRESS sets it apart from most adverse drug reactions. Symptoms may not occur for 3 weeks following drug administration. There may be a prodrome of pruritis, lymphadenopathy and fever. A morbilliform rash on the face, upper trunk, and shoulders is typical early in the course; skin lesions are present in the majority, but not all, cases. Periorbital and midfacial edema can occur. Multiorgan damage results in significant morbidity. The liver is most often affected followed in frequency by the kidneys and the lungs. Cardiac involvement (vignette 4) may be fatal and has been reported to arise in 4–27% of cases. An **eosinophilic myocarditis** can lead to necrosis, thrombosis, fibrosis, and even left ventricular wall rupture.

Diagnostic Studies.

- Extensive laboratory testing, including monitoring of liver and renal function status, to help determine the scope of organ involvement
- Complete blood count with differential usually shows leukocytosis with eosinophilia (but peripheral eosinophilia is not detected in all cases, even when endomyocardial biopsy confirms eosinophilic myocarditis)
- Quantitative PCR assays to diagnose viral reactivation
- In cases with cardiac involvement: cardiac biomarkers (elevated due to necrosis), echocardiogram (often shows left ventricular dysfunction), CT angiography (often unremarkable), cardiac MRI (detects inflammatory tissue changes and wall thickening) and endomyocardial biopsy
- Cardiac biopsy is not always performed. Skin biopsy may be useful to rule out other dermatologic conditions, including epidermolytic drug reactions.

Morphologic Features.

- Patchy myocardial involvement may result in biopsy sampling errors
- Microscopy: the eosinophilic myocarditis is characterized by a lymphocytic and eosinophilic infiltrate

Differential Diagnosis. Eosinophilic myocarditis can be caused by other noninfectious diseases and by microbial pathogens. Infectious etiologies include Coxsackie viruses A and B, *Trypanosoma cruzi* (South America), *Toxoplasma gondii* (exposure to domestic cat feces), trichinosis (consumption of pork products), and *Borrelia burgdorferi*. Noninfectious etiologies include eosinophilic granulomatosis with polyangiitis (EGPA). Blood cultures and antinuclear antibodies are helpful in ruling out other disease processes.

Treatment and Outcomes.

- Delay in diagnosis of DRESS may lead to irreversible cardiac injury and death. The **mortality rate is 10%**.
- Immunosuppression with corticosteroids and discontinuation of the offending drug are key.
- IV immunoglobulin therapy has been used in severe cases.
- In cases with cardiac involvement, ventricular assist device implantation, intra-aortic balloon pumping, and ECMO may also be necessary.
- Patients suffer a long convalescence, and many are treated in intensive care units.
- Patients are followed closely during tapering of steroid therapy; organ damage may occur over time and recurrences are possible.
- Patients who recover from DRESS often go on to develop **autoimmune sequelae** including thyroid disorders, SLE and autoimmune hemolytic anemia.

Physiology Correlation. The eosinophilic myocarditis associated with DRESS can cause myocardial necrosis, which causes electrophysiological abnormalities. Initially myocytes lose potassium; the decreased resting membrane potential creates a current of injury that can be detected by electrocardiogram.

Pharmacology Correlation. Drugs that have been reported to cause DRESS include allopurinol, amoxicillin, anticonvulsants, fluindione, minocycline, omeprazole, proton pump inhibitors, strontium ranelate, sulfasalazine, antibacterial sulfonamides and vancomycin.

Cardiovascular

Vignette 5

A 56-year-old-man with a 25 pack-year smoking history sees his physician with complaints of dyspnea and weight gain. Chest x-ray shows pulmonary artery enlargement and echo shows right ventricular hypertrophy.

Pathogenesis. **Cor pulmonale** refers to changes in the heart due to increased pressure in the lungs. Chronic hypoxia in the lungs causes pulmonary vasoconstriction (hence pulmonary arterial hypertension), increasing pulmonary vascular resistance and putting strain on the right ventricle, which causes right ventricular hypertrophy.

Clinical Presentation. Cor pulmonale usually presents with signs of right heart failure, such as jugular vein distention, peripheral edema, and dyspnea. Lungs may or may not be clear depending on the underlying pulmonary etiology (i.e. COPD vs. interstitial lung disease).

Diagnostic Studies.
- Chest x-ray
- Right heart catheterization
  - Pulmonary arterial pressure >25 mm Hg
  - Normal CO
  - Normal wedge pressure (LA)
- Doppler echo

Morphologic Features.
- RV dilation
- Enlarged pulmonary arteries
- Hypertrophy of the muscular media of the small pulmonary arteries and fibrosis

Differential Diagnosis. Pulmonary embolism can also present with dyspnea, which can also lead to right heart failure. These patients, however, would have risk factors (Virchow's triad) that make them prone to an embolism versus patients with cor pulmonale who have preexisting pulmonary disease.

Cardiovascular

Treatment and Outcomes.

- Oxygen
- Furosemide
- Dobutamine/milrinone
- Cor pulmonale is one of the leading causes of death in COPD patients

Physiology Correlation. Lungs are unique in that alveolar hypoxia causes vasoconstriction of the pulmonary vasculature (in order to shunt blood to other areas in the lung that can adequately exchange gas), whereas everywhere else in the body, hypoxia causes vasodilation to promote more oxygen delivery.

Pharmacology Correlation. Milrinone is a phosphodiesterase inhibitor, increasing cAMP levels in the heart as well as vascular smooth muscles. In cardiac muscles, increased cAMP causes contraction, but in smooth muscles, increased cAMP causes vasodilation because it inhibits myosin light chain kinase. Milrinone acts to increase inotropy and also vasodilates ("inodilator"), and thus it is used for pulmonary vasodilation in acute settings of pulmonary hypertension exacerbation.

Vignette 6

A woman brings her 70-year-old mother to the doctor, stating that she has been more fatigued and forgetful recently, and she has been complaining of difficulty breathing. Her mother has also had some "fainting spells."

Pathogenesis. **Cardiac amyloidosis** (CA), nonhereditary transthyretin type (ATTR), previously called senile cardiac amyloidosis, is a rare form of amyloidosis. In this form of amyloidosis, amyloid is deposited in the interstitium of the heart and causes a restrictive cardiomyopathy, but other organs are spared. Wild-type TTR is an amyloidogenic protein.

Clinical Presentation. The majority of patients with ATTR cardiac amyloidosis are age >70. Diagnosis is often delayed because patients present with nonspecific symptoms, such as fatigue, dyspnea, arrhythmia (causing syncope, as in the vignette), and infarction. Features of right-sided cardiac failure may be present. Associated carpel tunnel syndrome has been reported. Since other organ involvement is often lacking in the ATTR type, a high index of suspicion is necessary to make the diagnosis.

Diagnostic Studies.
- Liver function tests, blood count, creatinine clearance
- Serum cardiac biomarkers
- Electrocardiography
- Echocardiography
- Endomyocardial biopsy is gold standard for diagnosis

Morphologic Features.
- Gross examination: cardiomegaly and left ventricular wall hypertrophy
- Microscopy: biopsy shows apple-green birefringence under polarized light microscopy (Congo red stain)

Differential Diagnosis. Syncope can have a neurologic or a neurocardiogenic (cardiac syncope) etiology, and the initial workup is aimed at determining root cause. Cardiac involvement by amyloidosis can also occur in systemic amyloidosis (AL), and treatment for that entity is different so the distinction is important.

Cardiovascular

Treatment and Outcomes.

- Novel therapies include TTR protein stabilizers and RNA inhibitors to reduce TTR production
- Heart transplant is usually not a consideration given the patient's advanced age.
- Poor prognosis

Physiology Correlation. The QRS complex on EKG is indicative of ventricular contraction. In infiltrative processes such as amyloidosis, the amyloid fibrils accumulate in the myocardium, preventing effective conduction throughout the Bundle of His. This causes low QRS voltage. In the setting of "normal" left ventricular hypertrophy without infiltrative process, one would expect high QRS voltage.

Pharmacology Correlation. Digoxin worsens arrhythmias in amyloidosis (especially for the AL type) because it can bind to the amyloid fibrils and potentiate digoxin toxicity despite normal serum levels. Digoxin works by inhibiting Na^+/K^+ channels, which inhibits Na/Ca exchange and leads to increased calcium levels in the myocytes, eliciting ionotropic effects.

Cardiovascular

Vignette 7

A 19-year-old man sees his physician for a sports physical for basketball. He is slim and tall. Cardiac auscultation reveals a midsystolic murmur with click.

Pathogenesis. Mitral valve prolapse (MVP) can occur in **Marfan syndrome**, an autosomal dominant connective tissue disease due to a defect in fibrillin-1 gene on chromosome 15. In Marfan syndrome there can be an abnormally "long" mitral valve that is redundant and flips into the atrium during systole. This causes mitral regurgitation as well as the classic midsystolic click on auscultation.

Clinical Presentation. Most patients with MVP are asymptomatic, making the diagnosis challenging. Palpitations, lightheadedness and syncope may occur.

Diagnostic Studies.
- Physical exam findings of Marfan syndrome including tall and slender body habitus, arm span exceeding height, long arms and fingers, hyper-extensibility, and pectus deformities
- Auscultation: midsystolic click with murmur
- Echocardiogram: dilated left atrium (LA), low ejection fraction
- Genetic testing

Morphologic Features.
- Gross examination of valve: hooding of leaflets, enlarged leaflets, myxomatous degeneration
- Microscopic examination of valve: expansion of spongiosa with edematous tissue

Differential Diagnosis. Aortic aneurysm is another common cardiac manifestation for patients with Marfan syndrome due to abnormal dilation of the aortic root. However, aortic aneurysm causes a diastolic murmur from the aortic regurgitation, as opposed to midsystolic murmur with a click as in MVP.

Cardiovascular

Treatment and Outcomes.

- Aortic monitoring
- Avoidance of strenuous activity
- Medical treatment with beta blockers and ACE inhibitors
- Surgical correction of valve if severe mitral regurgitation
- Normal life expectancy with early intervention

Physiology Correlation. Squatting increases preload and moves the midsystolic click later in systole (closer to S2). On the other hand, standing from sitting position decreases preload and moves the click closer to S1.

Pharmacology Correlation. Beta blockers and ACE inhibitors not only decrease mortality but prevent remodeling of the heart, making them the treatment of choice for patients with Marfan syndrome.

Cardiovascular

Vignette 8

A 64-year-old patient with chronic kidney disease comes to the ED complaining of pain "all over my chest." He had recently missed dialysis due to vacation. Auscultation reveals a friction rub. EKG is normal.

Pathogenesis. Uremic pericarditis is a complication of chronic kidney disease. In patients with chronic kidney disease, toxins may inflame the visceral and parietal layers of the serous pericardium.

Clinical Presentation. Precordial pain is the most common symptom. Chest pain may be relieved by leaning forward. Heart sounds may be muffled. A friction rub is not always present in pericarditis, and it may disappear as the pericardial effusion increases.

Diagnostic Studies.
- High BUN (and creatinine)
- EKG: normal
- Chest x-ray: pericardial effusion
- Echo
- Blood cultures
- Pericardial biopsy

Morphologic Features.
- Gross examination of pericardium: roughened epicardium, adhesions, and loculations
- Pericardial biopsy findings: Fibrous tissue and acute inflammation

Differential Diagnosis. Hypothyroidism can also present with pericarditis without EKG changes. In addition to chest pain, dyspnea, and friction rub, these patients would also have other symptoms of hypothyroidism, such as cold intolerance, fatigue, and brittle hair.

Treatment and Outcomes.
- Responds well to dialysis
- Cardiac tamponade may occur due to effusion
- NSAIDs for pain reduction
- Around 50% may recur
- Surgical intervention: pericardial window, pericardiotomy, etc.

Physiology Correlation. Uremic patients can also present with anemia because uremia causes platelet dysfunction, making these patients more prone to bleeding.

Pharmacology Correlation. Although NSAIDs are first-line treatment for uremic pericarditis, they must be used with caution. NSAIDs can cause gastric bleeding, and uremic patients are already at risk for bleeding due to uremia.

Vignette 9

A 3-year-old boy comes to the ED with spots on the abdomen. His mother reports he has had a fever for a week. Physical exam reveals conjunctivitis, mucositis, and edema of the hands and feet.

Pathogenesis. Kawasaki disease is an idiopathic medium vessel vasculitis that most commonly occurs in young Asian children. The exact pathogenesis remains unknown, but it is believed to have an immune-mediated origin. Some data suggest genetic involvement, since those from Japanese ancestry and siblings of those who had Kawasaki are at a higher risk of developing the disease.

Clinical Presentation. The most common (and most important) presentation is fever of unknown origin for >5 days. Other presentations include conjunctivitis, mucositis, cervical lymphadenopathy, and maculopapular rash. In addition, other nonspecific symptoms such as nausea, diarrhea, arthritis, and rhinorrhea can be present.

Diagnostic Studies.
- Diagnostic criteria: fever for ≥5 days **plus 4** of the following symptoms:
    - Conjunctivitis
    - Cervical lymphadenopathy
    - Oral mucosal erythema ("strawberry tongue")
    - Rash
    - Extremity edema
- Increased ESR/CRP
- Echocardiogram
- Coronary angiography
- CT/MRI

Morphologic Features.
- Gross examination: thickened myointimal layer of coronary arteries; calcifications; fibrin thrombin in vessels with patchy necrosis and infarcts
- Microscopy: infiltration of inflammatory cells along with destruction of internal elastic lamina

Differential Diagnosis. Strep throat also presents with exudative pharyngitis with cervical lymphadenopathy and fever; however, patients with strep would not have ocular or joint involvement.

Cardiovascular

Treatment and Outcomes.

- Aspirin
- IVIG
- Self-limiting but coronary artery aneurysms may develop (especially with delayed treatment)
- Surgery (CABG)

Physiology Correlation. Kawasaki disease has a predilection for coronary arteries and can cause coronary artery aneurysm. Laplace's law states that the transmural pressure of the arteries is proportional to the wall tension over radius. If there is a weak point in the vessel wall (as is the case in vasculitis with destruction of metalloproteinases), the vessel is not able to adequately withstand the BP and thus the radius increases to decrease the tension in the wall, causing aneurysmal dilatation. The thinning of the vessel wall caused by vasculitis also increases wall tension (think of a blown-up balloon), which also causes progressive dilation of the vessel.

Pharmacology Correlation. Anticoagulants such as low molecular weight heparin or warfarin may be warranted to prevent thrombosis in the setting of coronary aneurysm in Kawasaki patients.

Vignette 10

A 3-month-old girl arrives at the ED with a seizure. Physical exam shows some light-brown patches on the left arm and a systolic murmur best heard in the apex.

Pathogenesis. **Cardiac rhabdomyoma** is the most common primary cardiac tumor in the pediatric population. It usually is associated with tuberous sclerosis.

Clinical Presentation. Presentations range from no symptoms at all to a murmur (as in the vignette), arrhythmia and/or infarction causing chest pain, or as an obstruction causing heart failure. Tuberous sclerosis manifests with seizures, skin abnormalities and with presenting signs of a benign tumor, such as cardiac rhabdomyoma.

Diagnostic Studies.
- Prenatal U/S
- Echocardiogram
- CT/ MRI

Morphologic Features.
- Gross examination: small, firm, off-white masses that protrude into the ventricle
- "Spider cells": large cells with cytoplasmic vacuoles

Differential Diagnosis. While benign cardiac myxomas tend to arise from the atria, cardiac rhabdomyomas tend to occur in the ventricles. Another common cause of seizure in the pediatric population is febrile seizure, which occurs in children age 3 months to 6 years. The seizure usually subsides after 5–10 min and is completely benign, with no intervention required.

Treatment and Outcomes.
- Cardiac rhabdomyomas regress.
- If complications occur, surgery is a consideration.
- Seizure control for tuberous sclerosis patients (see pharmacology correlation.)
- Everolimus for reduction of tumor size and seizure control.

Physiology Correlation. The tumor, although benign, can be situated near the left ventricular outflow tract and cause an obstruction. The obstruction can cause a backflow of blood into the lungs, causing left-sided heart failure.

Pharmacology Correlation. Everolimus is an mTOR (rapamycin) inhibitor that has shown to significantly reduce seizures in patients with tuberous sclerosis, especially those who are refractory to the conventional anti-epileptic treatment. It has both antiproliferative and antiangiogenic properties. One of its major effects is immunosuppression and thus should be used with caution.

Test What You Have Learned

1. A 52-year-old woman with chronic kidney disease presents with precordial chest pain. EKG is normal. Auscultation of her heart reveals a friction rub. Which of the following pertains to the prognosis of the cardiac condition suggested by her friction rub?

    A.   Recurrence rate around 50%

    B.   Cor pulmonale is a leading cause of death

    C.   Delayed treatment may cause coronary artery aneurysms

    D.   Heart transplant may be needed

    E.   Ranson criteria predict prognosis

    F.   Self-limiting due to tumor regression

2. A 3-year-old girl has had 3 days of fever to 39 C (102.2 F), conjunctivitis, swollen neck nodes, and rash extending to the trunk and genitals. What other finding is most likely to be seen with this child's condition?

    A.   Apple-green birefringence

    B.   Coronary artery aneurysms

    C.   Normal EKG

    D.   "Spider cells"

    E.   "Strawberry tongue"

    F.   Thinned, elongated chordae tendineae

3. A 5-week-old boy is noted to have an arrhythmia on auscultation. Ultrasound shows a 1 cm mass in the left ventricle. What other finding is most likely to be seen with this patient?

    A.   Arachnodactyly

    B.   "Ash leaf" lesions

    C.   Janeway lesions

    D.   Mucositis

    E.   Osler's nodes

    F.   Thumb sign

4. A 64-year-old woman with chronic emphysema is found to have jugular venous disten-tion, peripheral edema, and dyspnea. The desired treatment is medication that would increase cAMP levels. Which of the following would be the best choice?

   A. Beta blockers
   B. Digoxin
   C. Everolimus
   D. Low molecular weight heparin
   E. Milrinone
   F. Prostaglandin E1

5. A neonate who had appeared normal at birth develops severe cyanosis about 2 hours later. Lab studies reveal metabolic acidosis. Which of the following is most likely to be found on further investigation?

   A. Coronary artery aneurysms
   B. Dilated left atrium with low ejection fraction
   C. Egg-on-a-string sign on chest radiograph
   D. Hypertrophy of pulmonary vessel muscular media
   E. Large valvular vegetations
   F. Mass of the left ventricle

Answers: 1. (A), 2. (E), 3. (B), 4. (E), 5. (C)

CHAPTER 6

Respiratory System

Checklist of Processes Within This System

Developmental disease
- ❏ CCAM
- ❏ Bronchogenic cysts
- ❏ Pulmonary sequestration

Infection
- ❏ Nosocomial (hospital-acquired) pneumonia
- ❏ Lobar pneumonia
- ❏ Bronchopneumonia
- ❏ Empyema
- ❏ Fungal infections: *Candida; Cryptococcus; Mucor; Aspergillus; Pneumocystis; Histoplasma; Blastomyces; Coccidioides*
- ❏ Pulmonary TB: Ghon focus, Ghon complex, Ranke complex
- ❏ Secondary (reactivation) TB

Trauma
- ❏ Tension pneumothorax
- ❏ Flail chest

Vascular disease
- ❏ Pulmonary hypertension
- ❏ Pulmonary embolism

System-Specific Diseases
- ❏ Bronchiectasis
- ❏ Atelectasis
- ❏ DAD
- ❏ Pulmonary edema

- ❏ Diffuse alveolar hemorrhage: Goodpasture; idiopathic pulmonary hemosiderosis; granulomatosis with polyangiitis
- ❏ Chronic interstitial lung disease: cryptogenic organizing pneumonia; idiopathic pulmonary fibrosis; chronic eosinophilic pneumonia; desquamative interstitial pneumonia; hypersensitivity pneumonitis; pulmonary eosinophilia: Loeffler syndrome; drug & radiation pneumonitis; sarcoidosis
- ❏ Obstructive disease: emphysema; asthma; CF; chronic bronchitis
- ❏ Pleural effusion
- ❏ Pleuritis
- ❏ Transfusion-related lung injury
- ❏ Pneumoconiosis: asbestosis; Caplan syndrome; mesothelioma

Neoplasia
- ❏ Neuroendocrine tumors: typical carcinoid, atypical carcinoid, large cell undifferentiated neuroendocrine carcinoma, small cell carcinoma
- ❏ Lung carcinomas: large cell; squamous cell; adenocarcinoma
- ❏ Hamartoma
- ❏ Paraneoplastic syndrome
- ❏ Virchow node
- ❏ Pancoast tumor
- ❏ Carcinoma of the larynx
- ❏ Nasopharyngeal carcinoma

Representative Diseases

What follows are clinical vignettes for 10 select diseases within this organ system. First, read the vignette and try to identify the condition. Then, move on to read integrated information on each disease.

Vignette 1

A 15-year-old girl is hospitalized for a new onset of seizures. Once in-patient, tests reveal that she has a concealed pregnancy. She soon delivers a 1500-gram baby girl by emergency C-section. The pediatrician doing the neonatal examination notes tachypnea, nasal flaring, cyanosis, and expiratory grunting.

Diagnosis? _____

Vignette 2

A month after recovering from a viral upper respiratory infection, a 55-year-old woman visits her primary care doctor for treatment of a nonproductive cough. As he is taking her history, he notices that she seems short of breath. On examination inspiratory crackles are heard.

Diagnosis? _____

Vignette 3

A 60-year-old man who has never smoked begins to notice shortness of breath each time he mows his lawn. Over the following year, he develops a nonproductive cough. When his daughter observes that he sounds winded on the phone, she encourages him to see his internist.

Diagnosis? _____

Vignette 4

A 38-year-old mushroom farmer from Pennsylvania begins to have episodes of coughing and wheezing while working in the greenhouse.

Diagnosis? _____

Vignette 5

A 4-year-old girl is referred to an allergist for evaluation of wheezing and postnasal drip. Her mother mentions recurrent bouts of bronchitis, but there is little information about birth history due to adoption. On examination nasal polyposis is identified.

Diagnosis? _____

Vignette 6

A 40-year-old woman who has never smoked presents with persistent cough and recurrent pulmonary infections. CT shows a well-defined 2 cm perihilar mass.

Diagnosis? _____

Vignette 7

A 40-year-old man from Mexico presents with lower urinary tract symptoms and an elevated PSA. A prostate biopsy reveals granulomatous inflammation.

Diagnosis? _____

Vignette 8

A 45-year-old man is rushed to the ED after a motorcycle crash. He complains of left chest pain and shortness of breath. His blood pressure is 160/80 mm Hg, respiratory rate 28/min, and pulse 130/min. He has lacerations on the left chest and absent breath sounds on that side. His condition rapidly deteriorates.

Diagnosis? _____

Vignette 9

A retired miner presents with left chest pain and unintentional weight loss. CT reveals pleural plaques. A pleural biopsy shows spindled cells growing in sheets.

Diagnosis? _____

Vignette 10

A 45-year-old man is rushed to the ED for shortness of breath. He is known to hospital personnel as a drug addict, and needle tracks are present on examination. Chest x-ray shows micronodules throughout the lungs. On CT the micronodules are centrilobular, and there is dilatation of the pulmonary artery. An echocardiogram is ordered.

Diagnosis? _____

Vignette 1

A 15-year-old girl is hospitalized for a new onset of seizures. Once in-patient, tests reveal that she has a concealed pregnancy. She soon delivers a 1500-gram baby girl by emergency C-section. The pediatrician doing the neonatal examination notes tachypnea, nasal flaring, cyanosis, and expiratory grunting.

Pathogenesis. Neonatal respiratory distress syndrome, also known as **hyaline membrane disease** is a condition that occurs in premature infants. Premature birth disrupts vascular endothelial growth factor (VEGF) signaling, which is necessary for alveolar development. Surfactant production begins in the canalicular period of lung development and increases during the final weeks of gestation; in premature infants, type II pneumocytes do not produce sufficient **surfactant**. Surfactant reduces tension at the air-water interface in the lung, but it also plays a role in immunomodulation and host defense.

Clinical Presentation. The newborn normally has a respiratory rate of 40–60 respirations per minute; an increased respiratory rate (**tachypnea**) is the most common sign of respiratory distress. Other signs of labored breathing include grunting (as in the vignette) and intercostal retractions.

Diagnostic Studies. Chest x-ray shows hypoexpansion, air bronchograms, and ground glass opacities. Blood gas studies assess hypoxemia and acidosis. Complete blood counts and cultures are used to rule out infection.

Morphologic Features.

- Microscopy: lung biopsy shows eosinophilic hyaline membranes lining the alveoli

Differential Diagnosis. Other causes of respiratory distress include transient tachypnea of the newborn, congenital heart disease, infection, and meconium aspiration.

Treatment and Outcomes.

- Treatment includes antenatal maternal corticosteroid administration, neonatal surfactant replacement therapy, ventilatory support with continuous positive airway pressure ventilation (CPAP) and oxygen supplementation.
- The arrested development of pulmonary vasculature increases risk for **pulmonary hypertension.**
- Prolonged use of oxygen/ventilatory support causes retinopathy of prematurity and **bronchopulmonary dysplasia (most common cause of chronic lung disease in infants)**, and survivors have long-term airway obstruction symptoms similar to emphysema.

Physiology Correlation. Surfactant disrupts the surface tension of the water lining the alveolar surface. It is produced by type 2 pneumocytes in sufficient quantities for lung maturation by ~36 weeks gestation. Surfactant is primarily made up of proteins and phospholipids. Phosphatidylcholine is the major phospholipid. In respiratory distress syndrome, there is a lack of surfactant production and secretion. Infants benefit from surfactant replacement therapy. In adults, acute and chronic lung disease can alter surfactant production and content. For example, *Pseudomonas aeruginosa* secretes elastases that degrade surfactant proteins. Nonetheless, surfactant therapy has not been proven efficacious in adults.

Pharmacology Correlation. A course of **prophylactic antenatal betamethasone** therapy is given to accelerate fetal lung maturity in women at risk of preterm delivery. Corticosteroids accelerate the development of type 2 pneumocytes. Timing of therapy is key; infants delivered >7 days after antenatal corticosteroids have a greater need for respiratory support. Historically, when weekly doses were administered, fetal growth and head size suffered. Optimal timing and dose of betamethasone therapy are still under review.

Vignette 2

A month after recovering from a viral upper respiratory infection, a 55-year-old woman visits her primary care doctor for treatment of a nonproductive cough. As he is taking her history, he notices that she seems short of breath. On examination inspiratory crackles are heard.

Pathogenesis. Cryptogenic organizing pneumonia (previously known as idiopathic bronchiolitis obliterans organizing pneumonia or BOOP) is a pattern of lung injury due to alveolar damage. Organizing pneumonia may follow any number of insults, for example, infection, lung transplantation, radiotherapy and autoimmune disease. When this pattern of injury is identified with an unknown risk factor, it is called *cryptogenic organizing pneumonia*. There is no association with smoking.

Clinical Presentation. Patients present after a short duration (2 months) of a nonproductive cough, fever, and dyspnea on exertion. There may be a recent history of a flu-like illness.

Diagnostic Studies.
- Crackles on auscultation
- Lab findings not very helpful: elevated ESR and a leukocytosis without increased eosinophils
- Restrictive pattern on pulmonary function testing
- Chest x-ray: peripheral distribution of bilateral migratory diffuse alveolar opacities with air bronchograms, small nodules
- CT may show more extensive disease
- Open lung biopsy is diagnostic

Morphologic Features.
- Microscopy: lung wedge biopsy shows airspace granulation tissue (fibrotic polyps)

Differential Diagnosis. The diagnosis rests on finding the characteristic histology on lung biopsy and clinically excluding the other disease processes that are known to cause the same pattern of organizing pneumonia. Infectious pneumonia is the most common differential diagnosis. If the patient suffers from arthralgia or myalgia, a connective tissue disease may be considered instead. Chronic eosinophilic pneumonia (CEP) shares some features. Around 50% of CEP patients have asthma. CEP is characterized by alveolar and blood eosinophilia, and elevation of eosinophils in material obtained from BAL.

Treatment and Outcomes.

- Systemic glucocorticoid therapy
- About 30% of patients recover, but relapse is common upon tapering of steroids

Physiology Correlation. Respiration is controlled by automatic centers in the brainstem and by voluntary signals from the cortex. Dyspnea is a subjective feeling of uncomfortable breathing sensations. It is a perception of a need for greater effort to breathe, sometimes called air hunger. It is a common symptom among patients with chronic lung disease, but it also occurs in patients with cardiac disease. It is theorized that dyspnea arises from sensory signals.

Pharmacology Correlation. The use of systemic steroid therapy requires a balanced consideration of the risks and benefits. Serious adverse effects include diabetes mellitus, GI bleed, and bone fracture. An alternative treatment would be macrolide therapy for COPD. In addition to its antimicrobial properties, clarithromycin has an immune-modulating effect, partly due to inhibition of cytokine production.

Vignette 3

A 60-year-old man who has never smoked begins to notice shortness of breath each time he mows his lawn. Over the following year, he develops a nonproductive cough. When his daughter observes that he sounds winded on the phone, she encourages him to see his internist.

Pathogenesis. Idiopathic pulmonary fibrosis (IPF) is a nonneoplastic but fatal interstitial lung disease. While the pathogenesis is still unknown, recent research seeks to understand the association between gastroesophageal reflux disease (GERD) and IPF. The rs35705950 single-nucleotide polymorphism is associated with IPF. In 5–20% of cases, there is a family history of IPF.

Clinical Presentation. IPF is rare. It occurs more often in men age >50. A key feature is progressively worsening **dyspnea on exertion**. A nonproductive cough is usually described. Patients may show digital clubbing on examination. Bibasilar inspiratory crackles are heard on auscultation.

Diagnostic Studies.

- **High-resolution CT scan** shows reticular opacities and honeycomb change
- Pulmonary function testing shows restriction and a reduced diffusing capacity
- Lung biopsy shows changes consistent with usual interstitial pneumonia; in the absence of a lung biopsy, a diagnosis can still be made if clinical criteria outlined by professional societies are met

Morphologic Features.

- Microscopy of lung biopsy: patchy involvement of the lung by inflammation, fibrosis and **honeycomb change** (enlarged air spaces with fibrotic walls)
- Interstitial **fibroblast foci** (hypocellular eosinophilic collagen bundles)

Differential Diagnosis. Other causes of pulmonary fibrosis such as drug toxicity, autoimmune disease, and environmental toxins should be excluded.

Treatment and Outcomes.

- Survival is 2–5 years.
- Lung transplantation can prolong survival.

Physiology Correlation. Digital clubbing is a nonspecific but important sign in clinical medicine. A proliferation of connective tissue under the nail matrix gives the appearance of bulbous swelling of the ends of the digits. It may be seen in various serious conditions including lung cancer, IPF, and even cirrhosis. It is theorized that a circulating factor that is usually inactivated in the lung is shunted around the pulmonary circulation. First-pass catabolism of prostaglandin occurs in the lung, and systemic levels of prostaglandin E2 are increased in patients with clubbing.

Pharmacology Correlation. New onset or worsening of interstitial lung disease has been reported with biologic therapies, specifically tumor necrosis factor-α blocking agents that are used to treat connective tissue disease.

Vignette 4

A 38-year-old mushroom farmer from Pennsylvania begins to have episodes of coughing and wheezing while working in the greenhouse.

Pathogenesis. Hypersensitivity pneumonitis (HP), also known as farmer's lung, is an inflammatory lung disease with an immunologic basis. Some cases are the result of occupational exposure to aerosols including molds, bacteria, insecticides, and chemicals.

Clinical Presentation. The presentation may be acute or chronic. Acute manifestations include fever, chills, cough, chest tightness, and dyspnea 4–8 hours post-exposure. Symptoms of coughing often subside after leaving the workplace (as with the man in the vignette 4, who is sensitive to fungal antigens in the greenhouse). When antigen exposure is lower, symptoms such as dyspnea and malaise may persist over time with associated weight loss.

Diagnostic Studies.
- Physical examination is generally not helpful in making the diagnosis
- Chest x-ray shows bilateral reticulonodular infiltrates
- Serologic or skin tests for antigens may be helpful depending on the offending agent
- Material obtained from bronchoalveolar lavage is examined microscopically; a lymphocytosis is often observed but the findings are not specific enough to make a diagnosis
- Lung biopsy

Morphologic Features.
- Lung biopsy microscopy: diffuse chronic interstitial inflammation, peribronchiolar nonnecrotizing granulomas, foci of bronchiolitis obliterans

Differential Diagnosis. Wheezing, a symptom of asthma, is typically not present in acute HP. The finding of granulomas on a lung biopsy brings granulomatous infection into the differential diagnosis; special stains for organisms and cultures may be helpful to exclude infection. The granulomas of sarcoidosis are more tightly formed and occur along the lymphatic pathways.

Treatment and Outcomes.
- Avoidance of the etiologic agent (important for preventing irreversible lung damage)
- Systemic steroid therapy

Physiology Correlation. The cough receptors are located in the pharynx, on the posterior trachea, and at the carina. The internal laryngeal nerve transmits impulses to the medulla. The efferent pathway involves the vagus and the superior laryngeal nerve.

Pharmacology Correlation. Oral prednisone is a synthetic corticosteroid used for immunosuppression. Higher doses are used to treat acute HP. This therapy helps diminish symptoms but it does not change the disease outcome. The dose is tapered before the treatment is stopped. If exposure to the offending agent continues, irreversible pulmonary fibrosis still occurs.

Vignette 5

A 4-year-old girl is referred to an allergist for evaluation of wheezing and postnasal drip. Her mother mentions recurrent bouts of bronchitis, but there is little information about birth history due to adoption. On examination nasal polyposis is identified.

Pathogenesis. **Cystic fibrosis** (CF) is a common autosomal recessive genetic disorder. There are a multitude of mutations, and they determine the phenotypic expression and disease severity. At the cellular level, defective chloride and bicarbonate epithelial transport causes greater viscosity of mucus. In the lung, antimicrobial activity and mucociliary transport are impaired; repeated infections and bronchiectasis ensue. The exocrine pancreas, gut, biliary tree, and sweat glands are also affected. Cystic fibrosis transmembrane conductance regulator (*CFTR*) is located on chromosome 7. Most CF cases result from a deletion of the amino acid phenylalanine at position 508. There is autosomal-recessive inheritance.

Clinical Presentation. Most cases are diagnosed age <1 year. Pulmonary symptoms include recurrent upper and lower respiratory infections, coughing, and wheezing. Nasal polyposis may be the presenting finding in an undiagnosed child, as in the vignette. At birth there may be meconium ileus. Signs of malabsorption include growth abnormalities, vitamin deficiencies and malodorous stool. Most carriers of the gene are asymptomatic.

Diagnostic Studies.
- Prenatal, neonatal and postnatal genetic testing
- Sweat chloride test
- Imaging tests
- PFTs
- BAL and sputum culture
- Contrast enema
- Genotyping for possible therapy

Morphologic Features.
- Gross findings in lungs (autopsy series): mucus plugs and bronchiectasis
- Microscopic findings:
  - Hyperplasia of airway mucus-secreting cells, thickened smooth muscle
  - Pancreatic fibrosis
  - Steatosis and cirrhosis

Differential Diagnosis. Meconium ileus is not specific for CF; it can also be found in low birth weight infants. Hirschsprung disease is another cause of delayed passage of meconium. Because CF can cause wheezing and coughing, asthma may be another diagnostic consideration, but asthma can occur concomitantly with CF.

Treatment and Outcomes.

- Supportive care includes operative therapy for intestinal obstruction and gallstones, antibiotic therapy for pulmonary infections, etc.
- The FDA has approved the use of the small molecule drug ivacaftor for over 30 of the genetic mutations that represent a minority of CF patients; this treatment based on patient's genotype is an example of **personalized medicine**.
- Infertility may necessitate assisted reproductive technology after genetic counseling.
- Recurrent pulmonary infection causes significant morbidity and mortality.
- Life expectancy is improving and may extend beyond 40 years.

Physiology Correlation. CFTR is an ABC transporter-class ion channel protein. ATP-binding cassette transporters (**ABC transporters**) are involved in the transport of substrates across cellular membranes. Polymorphisms in ABC genes cause genetic disorders and multiple drug resistance.

Pharmacology Correlation. CF patients are susceptible to highly drug-resistant respiratory bacterial infections caused by *Burkholderia* spp. Single agent antibiotic therapy is not effective; susceptibility testing of isolates from respiratory cultures has shown sensitivity to ceftazidime combined with the non-β-lactam β-lactamase inhibitor, avibactam.

Respiratory

Vignette 6

A 40-year-old woman who has never smoked presents with persistent cough and recurrent pulmonary infections. CT shows a well-defined 2 cm perihilar mass.

Pathogenesis. **Typical carcinoid** is a subtype of bronchial carcinoid, which is a rare, pulmonary neuroendocrine tumor (NET) arising from the foregut. Typical carcinoid arises most commonly in a central location in patients who tend to be younger than other lung cancer patients and who lack a smoking history. Rarely there is a multiple endocrine neoplasia 1 **(MEN 1)** family history. *MEN1* encodes the nuclear tumor suppressor protein, menin. There is endocrine gland pathology associated with MEN 1 (the 3 Ps): parathyroid (hyperplasia and adenoma), pancreas (lethal functioning tumors), and pituitary (prolactin macroadenoma).

Clinical Presentation. Typical **carcinoid** is more common than **atypical carcinoid**, but both are less common than their counterpart in the GI tract. Some tumors produce symptoms (cough, infection, hemoptysis) but others are **incidental findings on x-ray.** Presentation with carcinoid syndrome is rare. Symptoms of **carcinoid syndrome** include skin flushing, facial skin lesions, diarrhea, dyspnea, and tachycardia.

Diagnostic Studies.
- Chest x-ray shows a round or oval opacity with a sharp margin.
- CT may show marked homogeneous contrast enhancement due to the rich vascularity of the tumor.
- Excisional biopsy is necessary for definitive histologic diagnosis.
- Lab tests if carcinoid syndrome is suspected: urine test (serotonin) and blood test (chromogranin A).

Morphologic Features.
- **Gross examination** shows a well-demarcated bronchial tumor bulging into the bronchial lumen.
- **Microscopically,** there are nests of uniform cells with clumped, open chromatin.
- Microscopic examination is necessary to distinguish typical carcinoid from atypical carcinoid (necrosis and a higher mitotic count).

Differential Diagnosis. On imaging, the differential diagnosis includes aspirated foreign body (age <5, right mainstem bronchus, M > F), pulmonary hamartoma (more common in the periphery), endobronchial papilloma (decade 5), and endobronchial fibroepithelial polyp (extremely rare and caused by chronic inflammation). Microscopically, carcinoids with a glandular pattern have to be distinguished from adenocarcinoma.

Treatment and Outcomes.

- Carcinoid tumors are grouped with other epithelial tumors with neuroendocrine differentiation. In the spectrum of pulmonary neuroendocrine tumors, typical carcinoid is low grade, atypical carcinoid is intermediate grade, and large cell neuroendocrine carcinoma and small cell lung cancer are high grade.

- Carcinoids are staged according to **TNM guidelines** and treated with **surgical resection** with surveillance for recurrence. Metastases occur most commonly in liver and bone.

- Other treatments include radiation, chemotherapy, and targeted therapy. **Somatostatin analogs** are not reserved for carcinoid syndrome; they have utility in controlling tumor growth.

- 5-year survival rate for typical carcinoid is >95%.

Physiology Correlation. The evolution of obstruction caused by a foreign body or endobronchial tumor can be explained by 3 mechanisms: bypass-valve stage, check-valve stage and stop-valve phase. In the bypass-valve phase, air may enter and exit; wheezing is the predominant result. In the check-valve phase, air may enter but may not exit; emphysema results. As the tumor grows or the swelling around a foreign body increases, the stop-valve phase ensues, and air neither enters nor exits. Atelectasis and pneumonia result.

Pharmacology Correlation. **Somatostatin analogs** have direct and indirect effects on tumor growth. These drugs directly inhibit tumor growth and induce apoptosis. Indirectly, they decrease tumor angiogenesis by inhibiting vascular endothelial growth factor (VEGF). **Tachyphylaxis** (rapid onset of a decreased response to a drug) ultimately limits their utility. **Cholestasis** is a common adverse effect.

Vignette 7

A 40-year-old man from Mexico presents with lower urinary tract symptoms and an elevated PSA. A prostate biopsy reveals granulomatous inflammation.

Pathogenesis. *Mycobacterium tuberculosis* is an aerobic bacillus that kills over 1 million people worldwide each year.

Clinical Presentation. Clinical categories of *Mycobacterium tuberculosis* disease:

- Latent TB infection: Asymptomatic, positive tuberculin skin test (TST), normal CXR and negative sputum smear, not contagious, may develop disease if not treated.
- Pulmonary TB disease: Symptoms of cough, hemoptysis, fever, night sweats, anorexia; + TST, positive smear and culture. The **Ghon complex** is a combination of parenchymal and nodal involvement. **Secondary** or **reactivation TB** shows consolidation with **caseous necrosis** in the apex of the lung; **miliary tuberculosis** (1-3 mm nodules in the lungs and other organs) is due to hematogenous spread of pulmonary TB.
- Extrapulmonary TB: Genitourinary TB is the most common form; it begins with hematogenous spread to the kidneys. Acid-fast stains of the prostate biopsy were positive for the patient in the vignette.

Diagnostic Studies.

- **Mantoux TST** is used only to **screen**; positive results requires further testing.
- False-negatives are caused by delayed-type hypersensitivity response, anergy, or infection with nontuberculous mycobacteria; false-positives are caused by BCG.
- Medical risk factors influence test interpretation; as clinical risk factors for infection increase, fewer millimeters of induration are necessary to interpret the result as positive.

Risk of Being Infected with Tb	Reaction Size Necessary to Interpret Result as Positive
HIV-infected persons; those with recent contact of someone with TB, with organ transplants, and with immunosuppression	≥5 mm induration
Injection drug users, children age <4 and all children exposed to high-risk adults, recent (<5 yr) immigrants from high-prevalence countries, mycobacteriology laboratory personnel	≥10 mm induration
Persons with no known risk factor	≥15 mm induration

Bacillus Calmette Guerin (BCG) is a vaccine made from *Mycobacterium bovis* that is used to immunize people in countries with a high prevalence of TB. **TB blood tests (IGRAs) are used to screen those who have received the BCG vaccine** and those who won't return for a second appointment. **In the analysis of pleural fluid,** an increased adenosine deaminase level ≥40 U/L fluid is suggestive of TB, cultures may be negative in >40% of cases; pleural biopsy is almost always necessary for definitive diagnosis.

Morphologic Features.

- Gross examination: **granulomatous inflammation** is the hallmark of *Mycobacterium tuberculosis*
- Waxy coat on the surface is impervious to Gram staining; **acid-fast staining** is used to visualize the pathogen

Differential Diagnosis. Pulmonary TB needs to be distinguished from **noninfectious granulomatous disease**, and parasitic or fungal infections (histoplasmosis/high endemicity Midwestern states). Congenital TB can mimic congenital syphilis and CMV.

Pleural effusion due to TB is **exudative**. Pneumonia, malignancy, and pulmonary embolism can also cause an exudative pleural effusion. **Granulomatous pleuritis** is almost always due to TB; rare causes include fungal disease, sarcoidosis and rheumatoid arthritis. On radiography, cystic tuberculous osteomyelitis has to be distinguished from eosinophilic granuloma, plasma cell myeloma, and metastases.

Treatment and Outcomes.

- **Latent infection**: regimens of varying combinations and intervals of isoniazid, rifapentine, or rifampin
- Factors determining outcome include host immunity and pathogen drug resistance.
- Drug resistant TB (DR TB) is increasing in incidence.

Physiology Correlation. Granulomas are formed by macrophages during a chronic inflammatory process. The presence or absence of necrosis in the granuloma is often a clue to the etiology of the disease process. TB granulomas tend to be associated with necrosis.

Pharmacology Correlation. To recall first-line TB treatment, use *RIPE*:

- **R**ifampin: orange urine/body fluids, increased metabolism cytochrome P450
- **I**soniazid: peripheral neuropathy, hepatitis not dose-related, drug interactions
- **P**yrazinamide: dose-related hepatitis, hyperuricemia
- **E**thambutol: optic neuritis

Vignette 8

A 45-year-old man is rushed to the ED after a motorcycle crash. He complains of left chest pain and shortness of breath. His blood pressure is 160/80 mm Hg, respiratory rate 28/min, and pulse 130/min. He has lacerations on the left chest and absent breath sounds on that side. His condition rapidly deteriorates.

Pathogenesis. **Tension pneumothorax** is an expanding air mass in the intrapleural space that can lead to cardiac compressive shock. Traumatic causes include a sucking chest wound or a pulmonary laceration. Occasionally tension pneumothorax is iatrogenic, occurring as a result of mechanical ventilation, acupuncture, subclavian vein puncture, or nasogastric tube insertion. Necrotizing bacterial infection (e.g., tuberculosis) can also cause tension pneumothorax. Sudden death may occur due to a precipitous drop in cardiac output accompanied with loss of ventilation on one side of the chest.

Clinical Presentation. Patients present with cardiovascular collapse and a **shifted trachea** with distended neck veins. If conscious, the patient may report symptoms of dyspnea and chest pain. Signs of cardiac compression include hypotension, tachycardia, and poor skin perfusion. **Neck vein distension** will persist while the patient is normotensive. It may not be possible to appreciate increased tympany over the involved hemithorax in the field if there is significant ambient noise. There are **decreased breath sounds on the affected side**.

Diagnostic Studies.
- Chest x-ray is diagnostic; findings include contralateral mediastinal shift; collapse of lung and flattening of diaphragm on ipsilateral side; hyperlucent ipsilateral thorax
- If patient is unstable, treatment of tension pneumothorax proceeds without x-ray confirmation of diagnosis

Morphologic Features.
- Biopsy is not performed.

Differential Diagnosis. In most cases there is no differential diagnosis. In the **setting of trauma**, the classic presentation often leaves little question about the diagnosis, and a diagnosis may be made presumptively on the basis of clinical findings. In the **setting of the intensive care unit** where the patient is already intubated, it can be difficult to recognize. The use of positive end-expiratory pressure (PEEP) may prevent a mediastinal shift; in this case, depression of a hemidiaphragm may be a more reliable sign on imaging.

Treatment and Outcomes.
- Needle decompression/tube thoracostomy
- Sudden death may occur if left untreated (due to decreased venous return to the heart)

Physiology Correlation. A tension pneumothorax occurs when a one-way valve occurs due to pleural compromise. Air is allowed to escape into the pleural space but not to return to the lung, leading to increased pressure in the ipsilateral hemithorax. When the ipsilateral lung collapses, breath sounds are lost on that side. The shift of the mediastinum kinks the vena cava and results in a decreased return of blood to the right atrium. Hypotension and tachycardia result.

Pharmacology Correlation. Depending on the clinical situation, during tube thoracostomy, local anesthesia is injected subcutaneously and in the muscle, periosteum and parietal pleura. Lidocaine has a rapid onset of action and can provide analgesia in minutes.

Vignette 9

A retired miner presents with left chest pain and unintentional weight loss. CT reveals pleural plaques. A pleural biopsy shows spindled cells growing in sheets.

Pathogenesis. **Malignant pleural mesothelioma (MPM)** is a cancer arising from mesothelial cells caused by **exposure to asbestos** in the shipbuilding, automotive, textile and asbestos mining industry. Exposure to the asbestos particles is also pathogenic in social contacts of workers. Germline *BAP1* mutations drive carcinogenesis. Chronic inflammation is an important component of cancer pathogenesis. There is a **long latent period** of decades between exposure and disease. The incidence is increasing worldwide. Mesothelial mesothelioma is less common than pleural mesothelioma.

Clinical Presentation. Given the association with industrial workplace exposure and the long latent period, most cases occur in men in decade 8. Symptoms include dyspnea; cough; pain inside of the chest/lower back; fatigue; weight loss, and fever.

Diagnostic Studies.
- CT
- Definitive diagnosis requires microscopic examination of biopsy material

Morphologic Features.
- Microscopy: tumor patterns are varied
  - Epithelial
  - Sarcomatous
  - Biphasic (combination of epithelial and sarcomatous)

Differential Diagnosis. Parietal plaques may also be seen in asbestosis. Microscopically, epithelial malignant mesothelioma may resemble adenocarcinoma; immunohistochemistry can distinguish one from the other.

Treatment and Outcomes.
- Surgery
  - Wide local excision
  - Pleurodesis (injection of an irritant into the pleura to prevent further pleural effusion by fusing the parietal and visceral pleura)
  - Pleurectomy and decortication
  - Extrapulmonary pneumonectomy

- Radiation therapy
- Palliative chemotherapy may be offered when tumor is unresectable at time of diagnosis, but mesothelioma is resistant to chemotherapy
- Targeted therapies are being developed.
- Median survival is 6–12 months

Physiology Correlation. The proposed link between chronic inflammation and mesothelioma begins with tissue fibrosis, which produces reactive oxygen species that cause DNA mutations with subsequent evasion of apoptosis.

Pharmacology Correlation. Trials are underway to ascertain whether aspirin therapy could reduce the chronic inflammation that drives carcinogenesis in individuals exposed to asbestos. Observational studies have already shown that aspirin may have a protective effect against colorectal cancer.

Vignette 10

A 45-year-old man is rushed to the ED for shortness of breath. He is known to hospital personnel as a drug addict, and needle tracks are present on examination. Chest x-ray shows micronodules throughout the lungs. On CT the micronodules are centrilobular, and there is dilatation of the pulmonary artery. An echocardiogram is ordered.

Pathogenesis. Pulmonary hypertension (PHT) is increased pressure in the pulmonary vasculature, specifically, **pulmonary artery pressure >25 mm of mercury (Hg)** at rest. **Primary PHT** is also called idiopathic PHT; a cause cannot be identified. Some cases are familial and disease occurs in some but not all individuals with mutations of *BMPR2*. **Secondary PHT** is caused primarily by an increase in blood flow to the lung; a decrease in venous outflow from the lung; damaged/occluded vessels; or vasoconstriction. The causes may originate within the lung or outside the lung. Valvular disease and heart failure are common causes of secondary PHT. Pediatric patients undergoing surgical correction of congenital heart disease often develop postoperative PHT.

Many diseases are complicated by PHT; PHT is a cause of mortality in bronchopulmonary dysplasia, chronic kidney disease and sickle cell disease. The patient in the vignette has PHT secondary to excipient lung disease caused by injecting crushed oxycodone tablets; the excipient in oxycodone—microcrystalline cellulose—causes granuloma formation.

Clinical Presentation. Coughing, dyspnea, fatigue, and angina.

Diagnostic Studies.
- Echocardiographic assessment
- CT angiogram
- Lab evaluation of coagulation
- Diagnosis is sometimes made by the pathologist when lung is biopsied for another reason

Morphologic Features on microscopic examination.
- **Medial hypertrophy of pulmonary arteries, intimal proliferation**
- Atherosclerosis of pulmonary artery
- When PHT is associated with injection drug use, clear or weakly staining birefringent crystals can be seen with H & E staining of the lung biopsy

Differential Diagnosis. Pulmonary artery dilatation can also occur in the setting of pulmonary fibrosis and due to a congenital anomaly that causes pulmonary trunk enlargement.

Treatment and Outcomes.
- The PHT changes of the vasculature predispose to embolic events.
- Treatment is aimed at the underlying cause in cases of secondary PHT.
- Supportive measures include supplemental oxygen, inhaled nitric oxide, diuretics and anticoagulants.
- Lung transplantation is a consideration.
- PHT can cause disability and death
- 5-year survival rate for pediatric PHT is 75%

Physiology Correlation. **Cor pulmonale** refers to changes in the heart due to increased pressure in the lungs. The right heart must work harder to pump blood into the lungs when the pressure is high. Consequently, the right ventricular wall may hypertrophy and heart failure may ensue.

Pharmacology Correlation. Nitric oxide (NO) is a selective pulmonary vasodilator that is used to improve oxygenation in PHT patients. It increases the intracellular level of cGMP. NO is toxic to platelets.

Test What You Have Learned

1. A 67-year-old man complains of chronic shortness of breath. The man has worked for 40 years in shipbuilding, where he was exposed to asbestos in his work. Medical evaluation demonstrates the existence of a pleural based mass adherent to his chest wall. Biopsy of this mass would most likely show which of the following?

   A. Airspace granulation tissue

   B. Biphasic pattern of epithelioid and sarcomatous cells

   C. Eosinophilic hyaline membrane lining alveoli

   D. Massively enlarged airspaces

   E. Nests of uniform tumor cells with clumped, open chromatin

   F. Patchy inflammation, fibrosis, and honeycomb change

2. A neonate who was born in the second trimester requires prolonged oxygen/ventilator support. This baby would be most likely to develop which of the following complications?

   A. Bronchopulmonary dysplasia

   B. Fibromuscular dysplasia

   C. Granulomatous pleuritis

   D. Tuberculosis

   E. Recurrent urinary tract infections

   F. Sudden death

3. An 8-month-old boy has experienced multiple bouts of pneumonia. The child was born at term in the United States. Chest x-ray shows early bronchiectasis. Which of the following would be most likely to establish this child's diagnosis?

   A. Blood chromogranin A

   B. Hypoxemia and acidosis

   C. Mantoux tuberculin skin test

   D. Serologic or skin tests for antigens

   E. Sweat chloride test

   F. Urine serotonin

4. A 35-year-old man is under treatment for tuberculosis that he acquired as a medical worker in Africa. He starts coughing and then he abruptly develops shortness of breath with chest pain and falls to the ground. Emergency radiologic examination would most likely show which of the following as a new finding?

    A. Bilateral reticulonodular infiltrates
    B. Contralateral mediastinal shift with lung collapse
    C. Dilated left ventricle
    D. Mass of the right upper lobe parenchyma of lung
    E. Pleural based mass of the left lower lung
    F. Reticular opacities and honeycomb change

5. A 55-year-old man consults a physician because of persistent shortness of breath, particularly on exertion. Pulmonary function tests show restriction and a reduced diffusing capacity. High resolution CT scan shows reticular opacities and honeycomb change. Which of the following would be likely on lung biopsy?

    A. Necrotizing granulomas
    B. Nonnecrotizing granulomas
    C. Birefringent crystals
    D. Round cysts in intraalveolar exudate
    E. Plexiform lesions
    F. Fibroblastic foci

Answers: 1. (B), 2. (A), 3. (E), 4. (B), 5. (F)

CHAPTER 7

Gastrointestinal System

Developmental Disorders

- ❏ T-E fistula
- ❏ Esophageal diverticula
- ❏ Esophageal atresia
- ❏ Hiatal hernia
- ❏ Gastric heterotopia
- ❏ Pyloric stenosis

Infections

- ❏ *Candida* esophagitis
- ❏ *H. pylori* gastritis
- ❏ Infectious colitis
- ❏ Parasites
- ❏ Necrotizing enterocolitis
- ❏ Viral hepatitis
- ❏ Food poisoning
- ❏ Amebic liver abscess

Inflammatory Disease

- ❏ Inflammatory bowel disease
- ❏ Irritable bowel syndrome
- ❏ Acute and chronic pancreatitis
- ❏ Appendicitis
- ❏ Cholecystitis
- ❏ Autoimmune hepatitis

Vascular Diseases

- ❏ Esophageal varices
- ❏ Budd-Chiari syndrome
- ❏ Hemorrhoids
- ❏ Angiodysplasia

System-Specific Diseases

- ❏ Obstruction: achalasia, intussusception, herniation, volvulus, adhesions
- ❏ Polyps: hyperplastic polyps, adenomas, familial syndromes
- ❏ Cirrhosis
- ❏ Primary biliary cirrhosis
- ❏ Biliary tract obstruction
- ❏ Primary sclerosing cholangitis
- ❏ Hemochromatosis
- ❏ Pancreatic pseudocyst

Masses and Neoplasia

- ❏ Esophageal squamous cell carcinoma
- ❏ Gastric adenocarcinoma
- ❏ Gastric lymphoma
- ❏ Carcinoid
- ❏ Gastrointestinal stromal tumor (GIST)
- ❏ Hepatocellular carcinoma (HCC)
- ❏ Focal nodular hyperplasia
- ❏ Pancreatic adenocarcinoma
- ❏ Cystic pancreas neoplasms
- ❏ Colorectal carcinoma
- ❏ Anal cancer

Representative Diseases

What follows are clinical vignettes for 10 select diseases within this organ system. First, read the vignette and try to identify the condition. Then, move on to read integrated information on each disease.

Vignette 1

A 42-year-old overweight man complains to his physician of intermittent chest pain occurring predominantly at night after he eats dinner or has a few drinks. The pain is mostly retrosternal and burning in quality and resolves spontaneously after about an hour. Vital signs and physical exam are all normal.

Diagnosis? _____

Vignette 2

A 38-year-old woman presents with chronic fatigue and abdominal pain, mostly in her upper abdomen and not temporally related to eating. Physical examination is significant for tachycardia and pale mucous membranes. Her abdomen is not tender and no masses are palpated. Labs reveal hemoglobin 9.4 g/dL and MCV 106.

Diagnosis? _____

Vignette 3

A 49-year-old man complains to his physician of epigastric pain. He has self-medicated with antacids for years, but never sought medical care. He reports loss of appetite and a 10-pound unintentional weight loss over the past month. Physical examination is unremarkable. Upper endoscopy reveals diffuse mucosal erythema.

Diagnosis? _____

Vignette 4

A 23-year-old graduate student returns from a semester abroad in India, where he did service work. His last project involved spending 2 days in a remote village. Several days after he returns home, he goes to the ED with fever and severe abdominal pain. He has not had a bowel movement in 3 days. Physical examination reveals hepatosplenomegaly and numerous pink-red macules on his trunk.

Diagnosis? _____

Vignette 5

An 85-year-old man with a history of celiac disease arrives at the ED from the nursing home. He is suffering from acute-onset, profuse, watery diarrhea. His temperature is 38.9 C (102 F), blood pressure 89/55 mm Hg, and pulse 118/min. Physical examination reveals diffuse abdominal tenderness and guarding.

Diagnosis? _____

Vignette 6

A 19-year-old college student presents to the student health clinic complaining of intermittent bloody diarrhea and rectal pain. She has never traveled outside of the country and has no sick contacts. Physical examination reveals a thin young woman in no acute distress with normal vital signs and no abdominal tenderness or masses. There is one area of perianal ulceration.

Diagnosis? _____

Vignette 7

A 15-year-old high school student is brought to the ED by his parents when he begins to slur his words. He denies any use of alcohol or illegal substances but reports that he has been feeling "down" lately and doesn't know why. Physical examination reveals fullness in the right upper quadrant and a brown ring around the periphery of his irises.

Diagnosis? _____

Vignette 8

A 42-year-old Caucasian man presents with severe itching for 1 month. He has a history of ulcerative colitis and underwent a total colectomy 5 years ago. Physical exam reveals linear scratches on his arms and back. The corneas are yellow and the liver is palpable 5 cm below the costal margin.

Diagnosis? _____

Vignette 9

A 2-day-old boy, born at 41 weeks gestation to a 19-year-old mother who received no prenatal care, has not yet passed meconium. On physical examination the baby is noted to have a large tongue, flat nasal bridge, low-set ears, and general hypotonia.

Diagnosis? _____

Vignette 10

A 3-week-old girl is born at 26 weeks gestation via C-section due to preterm premature rupture of membranes. She has been receiving baby formula through a nasogastric tube. Over the next 24 hours, she develops fever, progressive abdominal distention, grossly bloody stool, and bilious output from nasogastric tube. Crepitus is noted when the abdomen is palpated.

Diagnosis? _____

Vignette 1

> A 42-year-old overweight man complains to his physician of intermittent chest pain occurring predominantly at night after he eats dinner or has a few drinks. The pain is mostly retrosternal and burning in quality and resolves spontaneously after about an hour. Vital signs and physical exam are all normal.

Pathogenesis. **Barrett esophagus** is a metaplasia in the lower esophagus caused by inflammation. Chronic exposure of the lower esophagus to acidic gastric contents stimulates the squamous mucosa to undergo metaplasia to an intestinal-type mucosa. This columnar type epithelium is rich in goblet cells that secrete mucin, thus protecting the mucosa from the acidic environment. Untreated, **Barrett esophagus** can progress to dysplasia and adenocarcinoma. Risk factors include long-standing gastroesophageal reflux disease (GERD) and hiatal hernias. There is a significant male predominance.

Clinical Presentation. Patients with GERD often complain of burning mid-sternal chest pain, belching, or a sour taste in their mouth, especially after eating spicy or acidic foods or drinking alcohol or caffeine. Risk factors for GERD include obesity, pregnancy, older age, and smoking. Barrett esophagus is more likely to develop in Caucasian males, age >50, obese, and smokers. It is impossible to diagnose Barrett's without endoscopy and biopsy.

Diagnostic Studies.
- Upper endoscopy with biopsy of esophageal mucosa
- Both endoscopic and microscopic abnormalities are required for a diagnosis of Barrett esophagus

Morphologic Features.
- Gross examination: Lower esophagus shows irregular salmon-colored patches of mucosa
- Microscopic examination of esophageal biopsy: ***intestinal metaplasia*** = columnar epithelium with goblet cells filled with mucin (PAS-positive); dysplasia and intramucosal cancer may exist concurrently.

Differential Diagnosis. Peptic ulcer disease (PUD) causes epigastric, postprandial discomfort, or pain. Patients with PUD are less likely to complain of belching or sour taste in the mouth than patients with GERD. Upper endoscopy reveals a gastric or duodenal ulcer but normal esophagus. PUD patients often have a history of heavy NSAID use or are infected with *Helicobacter pylori*, which can be identified on biopsy.

Treatment and Outcomes.

- Lifestyle modification: weight loss and exclusion of spicy or acidic foods, caffeine, and alcohol from the diet to treat symptoms of GERD (**first step**)
- Proton pump inhibitors (PPIs) and H2 blockers such as ranitidine to treat and prevent persistent symptoms of GERD
- While overall risk of progression to adenocarcinoma is low in Barrett esophagus, the risk is higher if high grade dysplasia is also seen in the esophageal mucosa
- If Barrett esophagus is concurrent with high grade dysplasia, endoscopic mucosal resection (EMR) is a treatment consideration

Physiology Correlation. With stimulation from the parasympathetic nervous system, the esophageal smooth muscles contract in a series of waves called **peristalsis**. When food reaches the lower esophagus, vasoactive intestinal polypeptide (VIP) inhibits contraction of the muscles in the lower esophageal sphincter. This relaxed muscular tone permits entry of food into the stomach. In GERD, the lower esophageal sphincter is too relaxed, permitting gastric contents to flow backward into the lower esophagus.

Pharmacology Correlation. PPIs, which include omeprazole and lansoprazole, directly inhibit the action of the H^+/K^+ exchanger in parietal cells in the stomach epithelium. This antiporter normally moves K^+ out of the gastric lumen and H^+ into the gastric lumen. By blocking this exchange, fewer H^+ ions enter the gastric contents, thus reducing the acidity (increasing the pH). PPIs are used in the treatment of GERD, PUD, and *H. pylori* gastritis.

Gastrointestinal

Vignette 2

A 38-year-old woman presents with chronic fatigue and abdominal pain, mostly in her upper abdomen and not temporally related to eating. Physical examination is significant for tachycardia and pale mucous membranes. Her abdomen is not tender and no masses are palpated. Labs reveal hemoglobin 9.4 g/dL and MCV 106.

Pathogenesis. **Autoimmune atrophic gastritis** is an inflammatory disease of the stomach. Autoantibodies against intrinsic factor (IF) or parietal cells destroy gastric parietal cells, resulting in achlorhydria (low acid). Excess gastrin is secreted in response, which leads to endocrine cell hyperplasia. Because IF is required for absorption of vitamin B12 (cobalamin), chronic autoimmune gastritis can lead to macrocytic anemia, also called **pernicious anemia**.

Clinical Presentation. Many patients are asymptomatic until symptoms of anemia develop, but some patients may have epigastric pain. With long-standing vitamin B12 deficiency, neurological symptoms may include loss of vibratory sense and proprioception due to subacute combined degeneration of the posterolateral spinal columns. Like most autoimmune disorders, there is a female predominance.

Diagnostic Studies.
- Low serum pepsinogen
- High serum gastrin
- Anti-parietal cell and anti-intrinsic factor antibodies
- B12 deficiency may lead to macrocytic/megaloblastic anemia (MCV > 100) with hypersegmented neutrophils (>5 lobes per nucleus)
- Mucosal biopsy of gastric body required for diagnosis

Morphologic Features.
- Gross examination: Antrum uninvolved; body shows loss of rugal folds (flattened gastric mucosa)
- Microscopic examination of gastric body mucosa: lymphocytic infiltrate, intestinal metaplasia (goblet cells present in gastric mucosa), decreased parietal cells, increased enterochromaffin-like cells

Differential Diagnosis. Several other GI disorders can lead to vitamin B12 deficiency. Partial gastrectomy causes quantitatively less IF to be secreted; these patients are easy to identify based on surgical history. Terminal ileal disorders such as Crohn disease (CD) and fish tapeworm overgrowth cause reduced absorption of vitamin B12. CD causes skip lesions with transmural inflammation, fistulas, and granulomas throughout the entire length of the GI tract. Fish tapeworm (*Diphyllobothrium latum*) can be acquired after ingestion of uncooked fish.

Treatment and Outcomes.

- Management of autoimmune atrophic gastritis includes vitamin B12 replacement (see pharmacology correlation below). There is no specific therapy for gastritis.
- Long-standing vitamin B12 deficiency can cause subacute combined degeneration of the posterolateral spinal columns, which is reversible with vitamin B12 replenishment.
- Untreated chronic atrophic gastritis is associated with risk of gastric adenocarcinoma or neuroendocrine tumors.

Physiology Correlation. Parietal cells secrete HCl into the gastric lumen when stimulated by acetylcholine, histamine, and gastrin. To increase the parietal cells' capacity to secrete H^+, intracellular carbonic anhydrase converts CO_2 into $H^+ + HCO_3^-$. A luminal membrane-based H^+/K^+ ATPase pushes H^+ into the lumen, which increases the proportion of HCO_3^- inside the parietal cell. The HCO_3^- then diffuses across the basal membrane into the bloodstream, so the blood draining the stomach becomes highly basic.

Pharmacology Correlation. Vitamin B12 is the mainstay of treatment for megaloblastic anemia in autoimmune gastritis. The pharmacologic preparation is usually cyanocobalamin. By administering via the intramuscular route, it is possible to bypass the GI tract that is often the source of the B12 deficiency. Because there is no specific treatment for autoimmune gastritis, B12 replacement therapy is often lifelong.

Vignette 3

A 49-year-old man complains to his physician of epigastric pain. He has self-medicated with antacids for years, but never sought medical care. He reports loss of appetite and a 10-pound unintentional weight loss over the past month. Physical examination is unremarkable. Upper endoscopy reveals diffuse mucosal erythema.

Pathogenesis. **Gastric lymphoma** is a form of extranodal marginal zone MALT (mucosa-associated lymphoid tissue) lymphoma, or MALToma. Long-standing *H. pylori* infection causes chronic inflammation and proliferation of submucosal lymphoid aggregates that are not normally found in the stomach. If the infection remains untreated, these lymphoid aggregates can acquire mutations that lead to the development of lymphoma.

Clinical Presentation. Gastric lymphoma produces a multitude of upper GI complaints, including epigastric pain, nausea/vomiting, and anorexia.

Diagnostic Studies.
- Upper endoscopy with biopsy of the gastric mucosa is required to diagnose lymphoma.
- Biopsy can be cultured for organism identification and antibiotic susceptibility testing (see pharmacology correlate below).
- Urease breath test is positive (patient ingests labeled ^{13}C-urea, which is metabolized by *H. pylori* organisms. Patient then exhales labeled ^{13}C-CO$_2$).

Morphologic Features.
- Microscopic: prominent **submucosal B-lymphocyte infiltration** (CD20+) that may invade the overlying mucosa. ***H. pylori* organisms** (bacilli that stain positive with Giemsa or Warthin-Starry silver) may be seen within the superficial mucosal layer.

Differential Diagnosis. Gastric adenocarcinoma is an invasive epithelial malignancy that can also develop in a setting of long-standing *H. pylori* gastritis. Adenocarcinoma can present with a single irregular ulcer or diffuse involvement of the stomach termed "linitis plastica." Unlike gastric lymphoma, adenocarcinoma cannot be eradicated with antibiotics and has a very poor prognosis.

Treatment and Outcomes.

- Gastric lymphoma associated with *H. pylori* has a long, indolent clinical course even without specific therapy.
- Treatment with anti-*H. pylori* regimen eradicates the organism and the malignancy.
- With successful *H. pylori* eradication, relapse is uncommon and life expectancy is near normal.

Physiology Correlation. There are 3 phases of gastric acid secretion. First, the cephalic phase is initiated by the anticipation of eating by seeing, smelling, or thinking about food. In the gastric phase, filling of the stomach with food stimulates the vagus nerve to secrete gastrin-releasing peptide (GRP). In turn, G cells in the antrum secrete gastrin, which directly stimulates parietal cells to secrete H^+. Finally, the intestinal phase inhibits further release of gastrin by negative feedback as acidic gastric contents enter the duodenum.

Pharmacology Correlation. There are several combinations of medications used to eradicate *H. pylori*. Generally, they all include 2 antibiotics plus a proton pump inhibitor. Clarithromycin, amoxicillin, and omeprazole are a common "triple therapy." If the organism is clarithromycin-resistant on susceptibility testing, if regional clarithromycin resistance >15%, or if the patient is allergic to penicillin, metronidazole and tetracycline are used instead. Clarithromycin resistance develops either when the organism forms an altered drug binding site or develops a mechanism to actively transport the drug out of the cells.

Vignette 4

A 23-year-old graduate student returns from a semester abroad in India, where he did service work. His last project involved spending 2 days in a remote village. Several days after he returns home, he goes to the ED with fever and severe abdominal pain. He has not had a bowel movement in 3 days. Physical examination reveals hepatosplenomegaly and numerous pink-red macules on his trunk.

Pathogenesis. **Typhoid fever** is a form of enteric fever. *Salmonella typhi* is transmitted via the fecal-oral route, most often in regions with poor water sanitation. The organisms invade the intestinal epithelium and enter submucosal lymph nodes to gain access to the blood. Once bloodborne, the organisms can invade the liver, spleen, and bone marrow.

Clinical Presentation. Typhoid fever classically evolves over several weeks. Initially, patients present with fever. Over the next 2 weeks a skin rash develops with numerous pink/rose-colored macules. Hepatosplenomegaly, GI bleeding, and sepsis are other complications.

Diagnostic Studies.
- Blood culture and stool culture are positive for *S. typhi*. The organism produces H_2S gas.
- Gram stain shows **motile gram-negative rods**.
- CBC may demonstrate anemia and either leukopenia or leukocytosis if the organism has invaded the bone marrow.

Morphologic Features.
- Gross examination of intestines: prominent Peyer's patches (submucosal bumps)
- Microscopy: intestines, liver, spleen, or bone marrow
  - "Typhoid nodules" composed of clusters of macrophages with intracellular bacteria
  - Biopsy is rarely performed in clinical practice

Differential Diagnosis. International travelers may be at risk for other febrile illnesses associated with a rash. Dengue fever, caused by a mosquito-borne flavivirus, causes fever, severe headache, and diffuse maculopapular pruritic rash. It can progress to a hemorrhagic phase with bleeding from several mucosal sites, which is not seen in typhoid fever. Ebola virus causes fever, abdominal pain, and a maculopapular rash that becomes desquamative; vomiting and diarrhea are particularly severe and can lead to dehydration.

Gastrointestinal

Treatment and Outcomes.

- Untreated typhoid fever can lead to **intestinal necrosis and perfora-tion**, leading to overwhelming sepsis that can be fatal. Treatment should be initiated, even without positive cultures, for patients with classic clinical presentations and recent travel to an endemic area.

- Antibiotic choices include fluoroquinolones or third-generation cepha-losporins, specifically ceftriaxone. With treatment, the vast majority of patients recover with no lasting complications.

- This disease can be prevented by water sanitation and vaccination for residents of or travelers to endemic regions.

Physiology Correlation. Most nutrients are normally absorbed in the small intestine. Glucose, polypeptides, and amino acids are actively transported across the luminal membrane of intestinal epithelial cells via a sodium symporter. These nutrients are then passively transported across the basal membrane to enter the bloodstream. Lipids are broken down into fatty acids by pancreatic lipase, emulsified by bile salts into a micelle with a hydrophilic exterior surface, and diffuse across the luminal membrane of the epithelial cells. Fatty acids and triglycerides then enter the lymphatic circulation.

Pharmacology Correlation. Typhoid fever was formerly treated with ampi-cillin until widespread resistance developed. Bacteria can develop resistance to beta-lactams (including ampicillin) via 3 mechanisms:

- The bacteria can acquire the ability to synthesize beta-lactamases via a plasmid, thus inactivating the drugs;

- Structural alterations to the penicillin-binding protein (PBP), the target of beta-lactams, prevents binding of the drug inside the bacteria;

- The outer bacterial membrane can be altered, preventing entry of the beta-lactam into the bacteria.

Vignette 5

An 85-year-old man with a history of celiac disease arrives at the ED from the nursing home. He is suffering from acute-onset, profuse, watery diarrhea. His temperature is 38.9 C (102 F), blood pressure 89/55 mm Hg, and pulse 118/min. Physical examination reveals diffuse abdominal tenderness and guarding.

Pathogenesis. **Pseudomembranous colitis** (also known as *C. difficile* colitis or *C. diff*) develops from overgrowth of *Clostridium difficile*, a spore-forming, gram-positive anaerobe. The overgrowth occurs after antibiotic therapy alters the resident gut flora. The bacteria do not directly invade the colonic epithelium but produce 2 toxins (A and B) that damage epithelial cells, leading to inflammation and necrosis.

Clinical Presentation. Pseudomembranous colitis often develops after the patient has been treated with an antibiotic for another infection. Other risk factors include age >65, prolonged hospitalization, and residence in a nursing home facility. Clinical disease ranges from uncomplicated watery diarrhea to toxic megacolon, which can include fever and shock. If the megacolon perforates, signs of peritonitis such as abdominal rigidity, rebound tenderness, and guarding will be present.

Diagnostic Studies.
- Abdominal CT scan should be performed in a patient with an acute abdomen, and may demonstrate dilation of colonic loops indicating megacolon, with or without free air
- **Testing stool for the presence of toxin** is best way to distinguish active disease from the carrier state
- Nucleic acid testing (NAAT), while highly sensitive, cannot distinguish active disease from the carrier state
- Blood gas reveals a metabolic acidosis: pH <7.35 + low HCO_3^-
- Lower endoscopy can be useful if presentation is not classic (but is not performed if megacolon is suspected)

Morphologic Features.
- Gross examination: yellow patches ("pseudomembranes") adherent to colonic mucosal surface
- Microscopic: mucosal erosion, necrotic crypts, fibrinous debris, neutrophils

Differential Diagnosis. Norovirus is another common cause of acute, watery, nonbloody diarrhea that infects people living or staying in close quarters, such as nursing homes and cruise ships. This self-limited illness often causes concurrent nausea and vomiting, but not fever or signs of peritonitis, which helps differentiate it from *C. difficile* colitis.

Treatment and Outcomes.

- Metronidazole is the preferred antibiotic.
- Colectomy may be necessary to prevent rupture if toxic megacolon develops; megacolon is a poor prognostic indicator with high risk of death.
- Patients often experience frequent relapses after initial diagnosis whenever they are treated with antibiotics. Fecal transplant is a promising novel therapy.

Physiology Correlation. By the time food reaches the colon, only the electrolyte and water content changes. In the ascending and transverse colon, water and Na^+ are reabsorbed (water follows salt). An antiporter causes reabsorption of Cl^- while HCO_3^- is secreted into the lumen. Finally, K^+ is passively secreted into the lumen. Thus, diarrhea causes losses of K^+ and HCO_3^-, leading to acidosis.

Pharmacology Correlation. Clindamycin is the antibiotic most often associated with subsequent development of *C. difficile* colitis, but many other antibiotics have been implicated as well. Clindamycin is a narrow-spectrum bacteriostatic antibiotic that inhibits protein translocation in the bacteria. It is often used to treat cutaneous infections with gram-positive cocci, including both methicillin-sensitive and methicillin-resistant *Staphylococcus aureus* (MSSA and MRSA). In combination with doxycycline, it can also be used to treat pelvic inflammatory disease (PID).

Vignette 6

A 19-year-old college student presents to the student health clinic complaining of intermittent bloody diarrhea and rectal pain. She has never traveled outside of the country and has no sick contacts. Physical examination reveals a thin young woman in no acute distress with normal vital signs and no abdominal tenderness or masses. There is one area of perianal ulceration.

Pathogenesis. Crohn disease (CD) is part of the inflammatory bowel disease (IBD) family. IBDs are autoimmune in origin. CD can affect the entire GI tract, from mouth to anus. While the specific parts of the GI tract that are involved can vary from patient to patient, the terminal ileum is typically involved. This can lead to megaloblastic anemia due to malabsorption of vitamin B12 and steatorrhea due to malabsorption of lipids.

Clinical Presentation. CD typically presents with diarrhea with blood and/or mucus. Extraintestinal manifestations are common and can include fever, generalized abdominal pain, and oral ulcers. CD is most common in Caucasians, specifically Ashkenazi Jews, with a bimodal age distribution (adolescent-young adult and age >50).

Diagnostic Studies.
- Colonoscopy shows discontinuous areas of **cobblestone mucosa** with randomly interspersed normal mucosa (**"skip lesions"**), strictures (narrowing) and fistulas
- CBC may show macrocytic anemia
- Anti-saccharomyces cerevisiae antibodies (ASCA) are positive in 50% of patients

Morphologic Features.
- Microscopic: **discontinuous transmural inflammation** and **noncaseating granulomas** are the hallmark of CD
- Prominent lymphoid nodules under the muscularis propria are called "Crohn disease rosary"

Differential Diagnosis. Ulcerative colitis (UC) is the other type of IBD. UC is distinguished from CD based on the pattern of colonic involvement: UC causes a continuous ulceration and inflammation limited to the mucosa starting at the rectum and moving proximally. There are no "skip lesions." After colectomy, patients with UC are usually cured.

Gastrointestinal

Treatment and Outcomes.

- Inflammation in the ileum, present in most patients with CD, can lead to malabsorption of vitamin B12, leading to megaloblastic anemia.

- Transmural inflammation can lead to formation of fistulas, connecting loops of intestines to each other or other anatomical sites, including the bladder, vagina, and skin. Strictures may cause partial or complete intestinal obstruction, which must be treated with surgical resection of the affected area.

- Treatment options depend on severity of disease. Mild CD can be treated with glucocorticoids and oral salicylates such as mesalamine or sulfasalazine. Severe disease may require immunosuppressants, such as anti-TNF medications (see pharmacology correlate below).

- A relapsing and remitting course is common, but life expectancy is normal.

Physiology Correlation. Small intestinal epithelial cells have a number of channels allowing normal movement of electrolytes into and out of the lumen. Between the epithelial cells are tight junctions through which a small amount of sodium can enter the lumen. The basolateral surface has a Na^+ active transporter that secondarily brings K^+ and $2Cl^-$ into the cells from the interstitial fluid. Finally, the luminal surface of the epithelial cells contains Cl^- channels through which chloride enters the intestinal lumen. This channel is regulated by cAMP and is the site of cholera toxin binding; the toxin causes the channel to be constitutively open, causing massive efflux of chloride and water from the cells leading to profuse watery diarrhea.

Pharmacology Correlation. TNF inhibitors are used to treat CD and many other rheumatological disorders. Infliximab and adalimumab are monoclonal antibodies directed against TNF that interfere with the binding of TNF to its receptor. They do not have specific activity in the GI tract and can cause significant immunosuppression complicated by risk of infection. Before initiating an anti-TNF medication, it is important to test a patient for hepatitis B virus and tuberculosis to prevent reactivation.

Gastrointestinal

Vignette 7

> A 15-year-old high school student is brought to the ED by his parents when he begins to slur his words. He denies any use of alcohol or illegal substances but reports that he has been feeling "down" lately and doesn't know why. Physical examination reveals fullness in the right upper quadrant and a brown ring around the periphery of his irises.

Pathogenesis. Wilson disease (or hepatolenticular degeneration) is a genetic disorder that leads to copper overload due to an autosomal recessive mutation in copper transport ATPase on chromosome 13. There is decreased copper secretion and resultant copper overload. Ceruloplasmin, the copper-binding protein in blood, is used up to sequester the excess copper, making serum ceruloplasmin levels fall. Copper accumulates in many organs, including the liver, brain, and eyes, leading to a variety of clinical presentations.

Clinical Presentation. The initial presentation can be highly heterogeneous, with typical age of onset age 5–35. Patients may present with fulminant hepatitis, cirrhosis, hemolytic anemia, or neuropsychiatric symptoms including depression, dysarthria, dystonia, and frank psychosis. **Kayser-Fleischer rings** (brown rings around the iris) are virtually pathognomonic but present in only 50% of patients with Wilson disease.

Diagnostic Studies.
- **Decreased ceruloplasmin**
- **Decreased serum copper** (counterintuitive because the disease causes copper overload; the excess copper is bound to ceruloplasmin and not detected by routine methods)
- **Elevated urine copper** on 24-hour urine collection
- Liver biopsy to evaluate morphology and measure copper concentration in the liver
- Genetic testing to confirm presence of the causative mutation on chromosome 13

Morphologic Features.
- Microscopic: glycogenated hepatocyte nuclei, steatosis, and chronic inflammation. Regenerative hepatocyte nodules separated by bands of fibrosis indicate cirrhosis.

Gastrointestinal

Differential Diagnosis. Adolescents and young adults who present with acute hepatitis should be tested for the presence and concentration of alcohol and acetaminophen in the blood. New onset neuropsychiatric symptoms in this population could also indicate intoxication with other illicit substances that can be detected by blood or urine toxicology studies. Reye syndrome, caused by salicylate ingestion in children, can cause acute hepatitis with encephalitis; there is virtually always an antecedent history of antecedent influenza or other viral illness.

Treatment and Outcomes.
- D-penicillamine is first-line treatment.
- Liver transplant is a consideration if there is cirrhosis or fulminant liver failure not responsive to D-penicillamine.
- In the absence of severe liver disease, treated patients have a normal life expectancy.

Physiology Correlation. Copper can be involved in the formation of reactive oxygen species (ROS), which contain free radicals and cause significant cellular damage. In the Fenton reaction, copper or iron cations combine with hydrogen peroxide to produce the hydroxyl radical ($\bullet$OH). The hydroxyl radical then damages the lipid in the cell membranes, intracellular proteins, and DNA. This potential to cause major cell damage is why copper and iron overload states are dangerous.

Pharmacology Correlation. D-penicillamine is the mainstay of therapy for patients with Wilson disease (think "*copper penny*"). It is used both to remove excess copper that has been deposited in tissues and also to maintain appropriate copper levels in the maintenance phase. A copper chelator, D-penicillamine binds to the excess copper for excretion in the urine. Side effects include worsening of neurological symptoms and should be used with caution in patients with serious neurological manifestations of Wilson disease.

Vignette 8

A 42-year-old Caucasian man presents with severe itching for 1 month. He has a history of ulcerative colitis and underwent a total colectomy 5 years ago. Physical exam reveals linear scratches on his arms and back. The corneas are yellow and the liver is palpable 5 cm below the costal margin.

Pathogenesis. Primary sclerosing cholangitis (PSC) is a bile duct disease that damages the liver. It is likely an autoimmune disease, much like ulcerative colitis (UC), with which it is usually associated. With longstanding inflammation of the large bile ducts **(cholangitis), scarring and localized cirrhosis (sclerosis)** develop. This causes obstruction of the bile ducts, leading to buildup of bilirubin (cholestasis), and eventual jaundice, hepatomegaly, and possible end-stage liver disease.

Clinical Presentation. Approximately 75% of patients with PSC have UC, but only about 5% of patients with UC have PSC. Typical age at diagnosis is age 40, and men > women. Some patients with PSC are asymptomatic and diagnosed only when routine lab evaluation is abnormal. Others present with signs and symptoms of hyperbilirubinemia or long-standing liver disease, including jaundice, pruritis, hepatomegaly, esophageal varices, or ascites.

Diagnostic Studies.
- Elevated alkaline phosphatase, total bilirubin, and conjugated/direct bilirubin, indicating cholestasis
- Cholangiogram: large bile ducts show "beading" pattern
- p-ANCA positive in 80%
- Patient may be HLA-B8, DR3 type
- Liver biopsy

Morphologic Features.
- Microscopic: periportal concentric fibrosis ("onion-skin") centered around medium and large bile ducts. Overall loss of bile ducts. Hepatocytes are typically uninvolved and appear normal until late-stage disease.

Differential Diagnosis. Primary biliary cirrhosis (PBC) is another autoimmune cholestatic disorder which typically affects middle-aged women with autoimmune disorders (excluding IBD). Patients with PBC have a normal cholangiogram and biopsy shows granulomas, not fibrosis, of small bile ducts. Antimitochondrial antibodies (AMA) are typically positive.

Treatment and Outcomes.

- Ursodeoxycholic acid (UDCA) is the mainstay of therapy (see pharmacology correlate below).
- Cholestyramine can be an adjunct therapy for pruritus refractory to UDCA.
- Liver transplant is a consideration for patients who progress to end-stage liver disease.
- Without liver transplant, survival time from diagnosis is approximately 10 years.
- Cholangiocarcinoma develops in approximately 10–20% of patients with PSC.

Physiology Correlation. Secretin, made in the S cells of the duodenum, is secreted in response to entry of acidic gastric contents into duodenum. Secretin stimulates bile ducts to secrete HCO_3^-, which neutralizes the pH of the duodenal contents. Secretin also stimulates the release of conjugated bilirubin from hepatocytes to enter the duodenum. This water-soluble form of bilirubin helps form micelles composed of dietary lipids; micelles can then be absorbed in the terminal ileum.

Pharmacology Correlation. Ursodeoxycholic acid (UDCA), an exogenous hydrophilic bile acid, is often used to treat PSC. It is thought that UDCA sequesters hydrophobic bile acids, preventing their accumulation in the liver to reduce damage to bile ducts and hepatocytes. Cholestyramine, a bile acid sequestrant most often used to treat hypercholesterolemia, can also be used to bind and eliminate excess bilirubin in patients with PSC. While useful for treating pruritus, cholestyramine does not alter disease progression.

Vignette 9

A 2-day-old boy, born at 41 weeks gestation to a 19-year-old mother who received no prenatal care, has not yet passed meconium. On physical examination the baby is noted to have a large tongue, flat nasal bridge, low-set ears, and general hypotonia.

Pathogenesis. **Hirschsprung disease** (or congenital aganglionic megacolon) develops when fetal neural crest cells fail to migrate appropriately to the rectum in the first trimester. Ganglion cells normally stimulate forward movement of fecal material; when this motility does not occur, the portion of rectum immediately proximal becomes progressively dilated as stool builds up. Over time, the colon becomes massively enlarged (megacolon).

Clinical Presentation. Hirschsprung is almost always a disease of the neonatal period. It is usually diagnosed in newborns who fail to pass meconium in the first 48 hours of life, vomit, and/or have abdominal distension. Less commonly, mild cases may be diagnosed in older infants with chronic constipation. Males > females by 4:1. Down syndrome is a major risk factor for Hirschsprung.

Diagnostic Studies.
- Abdominal x-ray reveals colonic dilation and an absence of stool in the rectum
- Barium enema demonstrates a sharp transition from dilated to normal diameter rectum
- Rectal biopsy confirms absence of ganglion cells

Morphologic Features.
- Gross examination: massive dilation of colon proximal to affected segment
- Microscopic: lack of ganglion cells (clusters of large cells with large nuclei) in the muscularis externa; no overlying mucosal abnormalities

Differential Diagnosis. Another common cause of failure to pass meconium in the neonatal period is cystic fibrosis (CF). CF can lead to meconium ileus as the mutated chloride channel alters fluid content of the stool, making it viscous and difficult for the newborn to pass. Sweat chloride (the "sweat test") is elevated in babies with CF; many women also undergo prenatal genetic testing for CF.

Gastrointestinal

Treatment and Outcomes.

- Surgical resection of the portion of bowel lacking ganglion cells is curative; resection of the dilated portion of the colon is not necessary
- Outcomes are better in babies with short segments of affected colon
- Untreated Hirschsprung disease can lead to enterocolitis with fever and sepsis

Physiology Correlation. The colon is divided into segments called 'haustra' that sequentially contract to propel forward fecal material toward the rectum. Basal rate of contraction is controlled by the interstitial cells of Cajal in the myenteric plexus in the muscularis externa layer. As calcium enters the interstitial cells of Cajal, they eventually depolarize, stimulating contraction of the colonic smooth muscle. These depolarizations occur spontaneously throughout the day. As the colonic lumen fills, a "mass movement" coordinated through the length of the colon pushes fecal material into the rectum for defecation.

Pharmacology Correlation. Surgical patients are at risk for postoperative constipation or ileus for many reasons, including the use of opioid medications for pain control. A laxative regimen is often initiated when patients fail to pass gas or have a bowel movement within the first or second postoperative days. Senna directly stimulates the intestinal nerves to promote motility. Docusate promotes the reabsorption of water into the colonic lumen, hydrating the stool to make it easier to pass. These medications are commonly given together. Both may cause diarrhea as a side effect, and senna can cause melanosis coli.

Vignette 10

A 3-week-old girl is born at 26 weeks gestation via C-section due to preterm premature rupture of membranes. She has been receiving baby formula through a nasogastric tube. Over the next 24 hours, she develops fever, progressive abdominal distention, grossly bloody stool, and bilious output from nasogastric tube. Crepitus is noted when the abdomen is palpated.

Pathogenesis. Necrotizing enterocolitis (NEC) develops when the colonic mucosa undergoes ischemic necrosis. Prematurity and low birth weight are significant risk factors for NEC. The intestinal mucosa of premature neonates has not fully developed the tight junctions that normally help keep luminal bacteria from invading. Premature neonates also have immature immune systems, making them highly susceptible to bacterial infection. Antibiotic therapy alters the intestinal flora, which can lead to overgrowth of pathogenic bacteria. Breast milk may be protective against NEC in premature infants.

Clinical Presentation. Babies with NEC often present with a variety of abdominal signs: tenderness, bilious vomiting, and blood in the stool. Intolerance of oral feeding may be an early sign of NEC.

Diagnostic Studies.

- Pneumoperitoneum (air in the peritoneum) and/or pneumatosis intestinalis (air in the walls of the intestines) may be seen on abdominal imaging.
- Blood cultures detect bacteremia.

Morphologic Features.

- Gross examination: dilation of affected segment with dusky or hemorrhagic mucosa
- Microscopic: full-thickness coagulative necrosis. Adjacent but nonnecrotic intestine may demonstrate significant inflammation and edema with enlarged, pale cytoplasm.

Differential Diagnosis. Intestinal perforation can occur spontaneously in very preterm newborns. In these cases, imaging reveals pneumoperitoneum but not pneumatosis intestinalis. Bloody stool does not develop, which can also help distinguish spontaneous perforation from NEC.

Gastrointestinal

Treatment and Outcomes.

- Neonates with NEC are at high risk of sepsis.
- If NEC is suspected, broad-spectrum antibiotic therapy should be initiated, usually with ampicillin and gentamicin.
- Surgical resection may be required if rupture has occurred or is imminent. Long-term complications of surgery include stricture and short-gut syndrome.

Physiology Correlation. Carbohydrate digestion starts in the mouth with initiation of breakdown by salivary amylase. In the duodenum, pancreatic amylase continues the hydrolysis of carbohydrates into oligosaccharides. From there, a number of brush border enzymes (lactase, maltase, dextrinase) on the luminal surface of the small intestinal epithelium break down oligosaccharides into monosaccharides that can be absorbed in the jejunum (glucose, galactose, and fructose).

Pharmacology Correlation. Gentamicin is an aminoglycoside antibiotic often used to treat NEC because of its activity against gram-negative rods. Aminoglycosides inhibit protein synthesis by binding to the 30S subunit of ribosomes leading to translation of the wrong amino acid; thus aminoglycosides are bactericidal agents. Anaerobes are inherently resistant to aminoglycosides because the medications enter bacteria via an oxygen-dependent mechanism. Bacteria can acquire resistance to gentamicin via a chromosomal mutation that alters bacterial ribosomal binding site for the medication or by plasmid-transmitted ability to inactivate the drug. Gentamicin notably can cause nephrotoxicity and irreversible deafness.

Test What You Have Learned

1. A 42-year-old woman undergoes endoscopy. The stomach shows diffuse mucosal erythema. Biopsy of several of the erythematous areas shows dense CD20+ sub-mucosal to mucosal lymphocytic infiltrates. The disease process is most likely to be related to which of the following?

    A. *Candida albicans*

    B. *Clostridia difficile*

    C. Cytomegalovirus

    D. *Helicobacter pylori*

    E. Herpes simplex virus

    F. *Salmonella typhi*

2. A 3-month-old girl is readmitted to an intensive care unit with severe failure to thrive. She had been born at 27 weeks gestation, and at age 3 weeks underwent major surgery. Her weight is now at the 7th percentile for her age. For which of the following would her major surgery most likely have been performed?

    A. Atrophic gastritis

    B. Barrett's metaplasia

    C. Crohn disease

    D. Necrotizing enterocolitis

    E. Primary sclerosing cholangitis

    F. Wilson disease

3. A 37-year-old man with ulcerative colitis is noted by his gastroenterologist to have developed scleral icterus. Laboratory studies demonstrate elevations of alkaline phosphatase, total bilirubin, and conjugated bilirubin. P-ANCA is positive. Which of the following would be most useful in treating this patient's hyperbilirubinemia?

    A. D-penicillamine

    B. Fluroquinones

    C. Gentamicin

    D. Metronidazole

    E. Ursodeoxycholic acid

    F. Vitamin B12

4. A 7-year-old boy having difficulty learning to read is brought to an optometrist for evaluation. The optometrist notes that brown rings rim both of the boy's irises, and he refers the boy to a physician. Which of the following would be most likely to have contributed to the formation of the rings?

    A. Abnormal copper transport ATPase

    B. Acidic gastric contents

    C. Autoantibodies to intrinsic factor

    D. Fetal neural crest cell migration

    E. Poor water sanitation

    F. Premature delivery

5. A 15-year-old boy has been having bloody diarrhea. Colonoscopy demonstrates multiple areas with a cobblestone appearance in the cecum, transverse colon and sigmoid colon. Stricture of the colon is also seen in two areas. Biopsy of the involved areas shows colonic mucosa with transmural inflammation and non-caseating granulomas. Which of the following laboratory observations would be most likely to be linked to the patient's colon disease?

    A. Blood culture grows organism that produces H2S gas

    B. Decreased serum copper

    C. Megaloblastic anemia

    D. Positive pANCA study

    E. Ringed sideroblasts on peripheral smear

    F. Toxin is present in stool

Answers: 1. (D), 2. (D), 3. (E), 4. (A), 5. (C)

CHAPTER 8

Renal and Urinary System

Checklist of Processes Within This System

Developmental Disorders

- ❏ Renal agenesis
- ❏ Cystic disease of the kidney
- ❏ Medullary sponge kidney
- ❏ Prune belly syndrome (or Eagle Barrett syndrome)
- ❏ Pelvic kidney
- ❏ Horseshoe kidney
- ❏ Congenital vesicoureteral reflux
- ❏ Exstrophy of the bladder

Inflammatory Diseases

- ❏ Malakoplakia
- ❏ Interstitial cystitis
- ❏ Cystitis cystica and glandularis

Infectious Diseases

- ❏ Cystitis
- ❏ Schistosomiasis

Trauma

- ❏ Blunt renal trauma
- ❏ Bladder laceration

Vascular diseases

- ❏ Renal artery stenosis
- ❏ Fibromuscular dysplasia
- ❏ Hemolytic uremic syndrome

System-Specific Processes

- ❏ Nephrolithiasis
- ❏ Hydronephrosis
- ❏ Acute tubular injury
- ❏ Pyelonephritis: acute, chronic, drug-induced
- ❏ Acute postinfectious glomerulonephritis
- ❏ Hereditary nephritis (Alport syndrome)
- ❏ IgA nephropathy
- ❏ RPGN
- ❏ Nephrotic syndrome: minimal change disease, FSG, membranous nephropathy, MPGN type 1
- ❏ End-stage renal disease

Neoplasia

- ❏ Wilms tumor
- ❏ Neuroblastoma
- ❏ Rhabdoid tumor
- ❏ Renal adenoma
- ❏ Renal cell carcinoma
- ❏ Collecting duct adenocarcinoma
- ❏ Oncocytoma
- ❏ Angiomyolipoma
- ❏ Transitional cell carcinoma
- ❏ Sarcoma botryoides

Representative Diseases

What follows are clinical vignettes for 10 select diseases within this organ system. First, read the vignette and try to identify the condition. Then, move on to read integrated information on each disease.

Vignette 1

A mother finds an abdominal mass in her 3-year-old son. Upon clinical examination his blood pressure and other vital signs are normal. The mass is nontender. Genital examination is normal. Urinalysis reveals RBCs.

Diagnosis? _____

Vignette 2

A 35-year-old woman presents to the ED with dark urine, fatigue, and fever of 4 days duration. She states that she had bloody diarrhea a week ago, but that has since resolved. Physical examination reveals multiple red-violet pinpoint spots on her lower extremities and abdomen. Over the next 24 hours, her urine output decreases significantly, necessitating dialysis. On direct questioning, she admits to eating raw cookie dough 2 weeks previously.

Diagnosis? _____

Vignette 3

A 3-year-old previously healthy girl is brought to her pediatrician after her mother notices new facial puffiness. Last week she had a cough and runny nose which resolved spontaneously. Vital signs are normal. Physical examination shows periorbital and lower extremity edema.

Diagnosis? _____

Vignette 4

A 24-year-old woman sees a primary care physician to establish care as a new patient. She notes that her hands have felt "achy" for no reason over the last 6 months. On physical exam the distal and proximal interphalangeal joints are noted to be tender and have effusions. She has some sparse patches of hair on her head and painless ulcers in her mouth. Urine dipstick is positive for protein but negative for blood.

Diagnosis? _____

Vignette 5

A 61-year-old man presents with progressive fatigue and swelling in his lower extremities. Physical examination reveals fullness in the right upper quadrant, indentation in his tongue from his teeth, bilateral lower extremity edema, and conjunctival pallor. Urine dipstick reveals proteinuria but no hematuria.

Diagnosis? _____

Vignette 6

A 32-year-old woman presents to an urgent care clinic complaining of back pain and a low-grade fever of 1-week duration. She has a history of heavy menstrual bleeding with painful cramping but is otherwise healthy. Physical examination is significant for temperature 38.1 C (100.6 F) and an irregular firm, nontender lower abdominal mass. Urine pregnancy test is negative, but urine dipstick is positive for white blood cells and leukocyte esterase.

Diagnosis? _____

Vignette 7

A 39-year-old man is hired to help clean an old factory that used to manufacture industrial solvents. A coworker accidentally kicks over an unlabeled canister, spilling the sweet-smelling liquid contents. The man starts coughing within 30 minutes and develops a fever 2 hours later, prompting him to go to the ED. The next day, his urine output has decreased and the urine appears dark.

Diagnosis? _____

Vignette 8

A 22-year-old student presents to the health clinic complaining of headaches. She attributed them to stress from studying but they have persisted for several months. Physical examination reveals blood pressure 165/95 mm Hg. She denies smoking. She eats a vegetarian diet and exercises 4 days per week.

Diagnosis? _____

Vignette 9

A 27-year-old man presents to the ED with acute onset flank pain and blood in his urine. Physical examination reveals no abdominal or genital abnormalities. Exam reveals multiple oval-shaped pale macules on his trunk, multiple erythematous papules on his cheeks, and smooth, firm nodules protruding from multiple fingernail beds.

Diagnosis? _____

Vignette 10

A 19-year-old college student travels to Egypt during spring break. On a hot day she swims in a river for several hours. A few weeks after returning home, she notices blood in her urine. She denies any new sexual partners, dysuria, increased urination, or vaginal discharge.

Diagnosis? _____

Vignette 1

A mother finds an abdominal mass in her 3-year-old son. Upon clinical examination his blood pressure and other vital signs are normal. The mass is nontender. Genital examination is normal. Urinalysis reveals RBCs.

Pathogenesis. **Wilms tumor (or nephroblastoma)** is caused by genetic mutation in a tumor suppressor gene, most often the *WT-1* or *p53* gene. In a minority of patients, Wilms tumor may be associated with **WAGR syndrome** (germline *WT-1* mutation; **W**ilms tumor, **A**niridia, **G**enital anomalies, and mental **R**etardation) or **Beckwith-Wiedemann syndrome** (germline *WT-2* mutation; neonatal hypoglycemia, macroglossia, macrosomia, ear abnormalities, midline abdominal defects).

Clinical Presentation. Most children with Wilms tumor present age 2–5 and almost never after age 10. Other than the abdominal mass, they are often asymptomatic. A minority of patients have hematuria or abdominal tenderness.

Diagnostic Studies.

- Abdominal imaging (U/S, CT scan, or MRI) localizes the mass to the kidney and determines whether the mass can be surgically resected
- Chest and pelvic imaging are performed to rule out metastatic disease
- Biopsy of the mass is required for definitive diagnosis

Morphologic Features.

- Gross examination: large, solitary, tan mass in kidney
- Microscopic: triphasic morphology with glandular epithelium (resembling renal tubules and/or glomeruli), blastema (small hyperchromatic blue cells arranged in sheets, cords, or nodules), and stroma. The presence of anaplasia (enlarged hyperchromatic nuclei, atypical mitotic figures) in any of the components is a poor prognostic factor

Differential Diagnosis. Neuroblastoma is another pediatric renal tumor; it may be associated with elevated urine catecholamines and hypertension, which are absent in Wilms tumor patients. Microscopically, neuroblastoma demonstrates neuroendocrine features (rosette architecture, salt-and-pepper nuclei).

Renal and Urinary

Treatment and Outcomes.

- Excellent prognosis with surgery plus chemotherapy and/or radiation; approximately 90% 5-year survival
- Tumor spillage during surgical resection imparts a worse prognosis
- Children receiving radiation may be at risk for secondary malignancies in adulthood

Physiology Correlation. Mutations in tumor suppressor genes and proto-oncogenes are often implicated in oncogenesis. Normally, tumor suppressor genes such as *TP53, RB*, and *BRCA1/2* inhibit proliferation of damaged cells. Hereditary or acquired loss-of-function mutations of both alleles of a gene allow the development of malignancy (two-hit hypothesis). Proto-oncogenes are involved with normal cellular growth and development. A gain-of-function mutation converts a proto-oncogene into an oncogene that enables unchecked cellular proliferation. Only one mutated oncogene is required to promote oncogenesis.

Pharmacology Correlation. Vincristine is a chemotherapeutic agent used to treat Wilms tumors and many other malignancies. Vincristine binds to microtubules in the M phase of mitosis, preventing the formation of spindles. In addition to causing bone marrow suppression like most chemotherapeutics, vincristine can also cause peripheral neuropathy and neuralgias.

Renal and Urinary

Vignette 2

A 35-year-old woman presents to the ED with dark urine, fatigue, and fever of 4 days duration. She states that she had bloody diarrhea a week ago, but that has since resolved. Physical examination reveals multiple red-violet pinpoint spots on her lower extremities and abdomen. Over the next 24 hours, her urine output decreases significantly, necessitating dialysis. On direct questioning, she admits to eating raw cookie dough 2 weeks previously.

Pathogenesis. **Hemolytic uremic syndrome** (HUS) is almost always caused by *E. coli* O157:H7, also called "enterohemorrhagic" *E. coli* (EHEC) or Shiga toxin–producing *E. coli* (STEC), which secretes a Shiga-like toxin (SLT or "verotoxin"). This exotoxin inhibits protein synthesis by attacking ribosomal 60S in endothelial cells, particularly targeting the kidneys. As a result, microthrombi form in the small blood vessels of the kidneys (see physiology correlate below). There is a rare subtype called "atypical HUS" that is caused by complement dysregulation rather than *E. coli*; these patients do not have antecedent diarrhea.

Clinical Presentation. HUS often affects children but can occur in patients of any age. Patients present with severe abdominal pain, bloody diarrhea, and dark or grossly bloody urine with decreased urine output (oliguria or anuria). There is often a history of recent exposure to farm animals or petting zoos, or consumption of unpasteurized raw meat or eggs (vignette 2), which can lead to infection with *E. coli*.

Diagnostic Studies.
- CBC shows anemia and thrombocytopenia. Schistocytes may be seen on peripheral blood smear
- Markedly elevated BUN/Cr with hematuria
- Stool evaluation for SLT or culture for EHEC (however, may be negative by the time HUS develops because diarrhea has usually resolved by then)
- ADAMTS13 activity is normal (ruling out thrombotic thrombocytopenic purpura [TTP])

Morphologic Features.
- Microscopic: thrombi composed of fibrin and platelets in glomeruli and small blood vessels
- Schistocytes can be seen on peripheral blood smear in any microangiopathic hemolytic anemia (MAHA)

Differential Diagnosis. Disseminated intravascular coagulation (DIC) is associated with many systemic disorders including sepsis and obstetrical complications; PT and PTT are prolonged, fibrinogen is low, and D-dimers are high. Hypertensive crisis, or malignant hypertension, is diagnosed when BP >180/120 mm Hg and there are signs of end-organ damage. TTP is confirmed by identifying severe ADAMTS13 deficiency due to autoantibodies directed against the protein. Other infectious colitides can also cause bloody diarrhea and acute kidney injury from dehydration, but do not cause anemia and thrombocytopenia.

Treatment and Outcomes.
- Treatment is primarily supportive and involves fluid resuscitation and dialysis
- Antibiotics do not prevent progression of GI EHEC infection to HUS
- Overall prognosis is excellent, with <5% mortality rate

Physiology Correlation. HUS is a thrombotic microangiopathy (TMA), a category of disorders in which red blood cells lyse as they pass through the diseased small blood vessels. The resultant anemia is referred to as a MAHA and schistocytes (fragmented red blood cells) can be seen on peripheral blood smear. Because of intravascular hemolysis, hyperbilirubinemia with elevated direct/unconjugated bilirubin develops. Free hemoglobin released from the hemolyzed red blood cells is highly nephrotoxic, leading to acute kidney injury.

Pharmacology Correlation. Chronic kidney disease is the most common cause of hyperphosphatemia. While dietary limitation of phosphate should be attempted first, phosphate binders such as sevelamer are initiated in patients with persistent hyperphosphatemia. Sevelamer is a polymer that acts in the intestinal lumen, selectively binding to and inhibiting the absorption of phosphate. Calcium carbonate can also be used as a phosphate binder but is not first-line treatment due to the risk of hypercalcemia.

Renal and Urinary

Vignette 3

> A 3-year-old previously healthy girl is brought to her pediatrician after her mother notices new facial puffiness. Last week she had a cough and runny nose which resolved spontaneously. Vital signs are normal. Physical examination shows periorbital and lower extremity edema.

Pathogenesis. **Minimal change disease** (also called nil disease or "lipoid nephrosis") is a glomerular disease that causes nephrotic syndrome. Glomerular podocyte foot processes normally act to prevent passage of large molecules, such as proteins, from the blood into the urine. In minimal change disease, the glomerular podocyte foot processes are lost, allowing proteins to enter the urine. Loss of albumin, the primary oncotic force in the blood, causes leakage of fluid into extravascular spaces causing edema. To compensate for loss of plasma oncotic pressure, the liver increases production of lipids with resultant hyperlipidemia. The vast majority of cases of minimal change disease are idiopathic, but occasional cases are associated with Hodgkin lymphoma.

Clinical Presentation. Minimal change disease causes approximately 90% of nephrotic syndrome in children in the United States. Most affected children are age 2–6 years.

Diagnostic Studies.
- Nephrotic-range proteinuria, >3.5 g/day
- Hypoalbuminemia, hyperlipidemia
- Normal BUN/creatinine
- Renal biopsy is rarely performed in clinical practice

Morphologic Features.
- Microscopy: normal glomerulus
- Electron microscopy: **effacement/loss of podocytes** (epithelial cell foot processes)

Differential Diagnosis. Focal segmental glomerulosclerosis (FSGS) is another common cause of nephrotic syndrome. However, nearly all FSGS patients are adults, not children. On renal biopsy, FSGS demonstrates scarring (sclerosis) in portions of some glomeruli (segmental) with other normal glomeruli (focal).

Treatment and Outcomes.

- Because the majority of children with nephrotic syndrome have minimal change disease, empiric steroid therapy with prednisone is often started even without a renal biopsy to confirm the diagnosis.
- Vast majority of children have a full recovery with no long-term sequelae.

Physiology Correlation. Glomerular filtration rate (GFR)—the amount of fluid filtered in Bowman's capsule of the glomerulus in a given period of time—is often used to approximate renal function. Clinically, a normal GFR indicates good renal function while a low, or declining, GFR indicates poor or worsening renal function. GFR estimates can be made by measuring the clearance of inulin, which is freely filtered but neither reabsorbed nor secreted; there is a proportional increase in inulin clearance as plasma concentration increases.

Pharmacology Correlation. Prednisone, a corticosteroid, is used in the treatment of many inflammatory and autoimmune disorders. Steroids act via cellular and biochemical pathways. There is reduced capillary permeability, which reduces localized swelling, and reduced migration of white blood cells to the inflamed site, which prevents propagation of the inflammatory response. Steroids reduce the production of prostaglandins, leukotrienes, and interleukins, all of which promote inflammation. There are a multitude of side effects associated with long-term use, including muscle wasting, skin thinning, hyperglycemia, and osteoporosis.

Renal and Urinary

Vignette 4

A 24-year-old woman sees a primary care physician to establish care as a new patient. She notes that her hands have felt "achy" for no reason over the last 6 months. On physical exam the distal and proximal interphalangeal joints are noted to be tender and have effusions. She has some sparse patches of hair on her head and painless ulcers in her mouth. Urine dipstick is positive for protein but negative for blood.

Pathogenesis. Lupus nephritis is inflammation of the kidney caused by systemic lupus erythematosus. It is a type III hypersensitivity reaction in which antibodies bind antigens in the blood and subsequently deposit immune complexes in the subendothelium of glomeruli. Protein and blood can then enter the urine through the breached glomerular barriers.

Clinical Presentation. Systemic lupus erythematosus (SLE) occurs more often in women, mean age 20–45, with blacks and Hispanics affected more than whites. SLE is a highly heterogeneous chronic disorder. Despite the variability in clinical presentation, most patients demonstrate involvement of the kidneys at some point in their life, often at initial diagnosis. Patients with lupus nephritis can be asymptomatic, diagnosed only on routine lab evaluation, or may present with signs of acute kidney injury including dark urine and/or reduced urine output.

Diagnostic Studies.
- Proteinuria (nephritic- or nephrotic-range) with or without hematuria
- Urine sediment may reveal casts indicating active nephritis
- Elevated BUN/creatinine, reduced eGFR
- Autoantibodies: ANA, anti-Sm, anti-double stranded DNA (dsDNA) are usually positive in SLE
- Renal biopsy is required for classification

Morphologic Features.
- Microscopic: varies by class
  - Class I: ("minimal mesangial") mesangial immune complex deposition not visible by light microscopy
  - Class II mesangial: hypercellular mesangium
  - Class III focal nephritis: <50% of glomeruli show acute and/or chronic inflammation in a portion of the glomerulus

- – Class IV diffuse nephritis: >50% of glomeruli show acute and/or chronic inflammation in a portion of the glomerulus. Occasional thick-walled glomerular capillary loops ("wire loops") and crescents may be seen.
- – Class V membranous nephritis: diffuse thick-walled glomerular capillary loops
- – Class VI scarring/sclerosis: >90% of glomeruli are sclerotic/scarred
- Immunofluorescence: IgG, IgA, IgM, C3, C1a stains are all positive ("full house" pattern) due to immune complex deposition
- Electron microscopy: subendothelial electron-dense deposits

Differential Diagnosis. Poststreptococcal glomerulonephritis also demonstrates subendothelial deposits on electron microscopy.

Treatment and Outcomes.

- Steroids and other immunosuppressive medications are mainstay of therapy
- Many patients progress to chronic renal failure and dialysis-dependence
- Mortality rates are worse in those with nephritis than those without (only exception is those with pure class V lupus nephritis, who have a better prognosis)
- Regular urinalysis to monitor all SLE patients for proteinuria and possible lupus nephritis

Physiology Correlation. Class III hypersensitivity disorders are characterized by the binding of antibodies and antigens in blood with subsequent deposition of these immune complexes in tissue. This deposition attracts neutrophils, resulting in activation of complement and direct damage to local vascular endothelium. Type III hypersensitivity in SLE can cause arthritis or cutaneous vasculitis with palpable purpura. Some medications, including penicillin and monoclonal antibodies (ending in -mab) can cause type III hypersensitivity reactions.

Pharmacology Correlation. Mycophenolate mofetil is often used to treat SLE and lupus nephritis. By directly inhibiting the enzyme inosine monophosphate dehydrogenase (IMPDH), the synthesis of adenine and guanine (purine nucleotides) and subsequently DNA synthesis in lymphocytes is inhibited. Mycophenolate is teratogenic and can cause pregnancy loss, and should be used with caution in women of childbearing potential.

Renal and Urinary

Vignette 5

A 61-year-old man presents with progressive fatigue and swelling in his lower extremities. Physical examination reveals fullness in the right upper quadrant, indentation in his tongue from his teeth, bilateral lower extremity edema, and conjunctival pallor. Urine dipstick reveals proteinuria but no hematuria.

Pathogenesis. **Renal amyloidosis** is a potentially life-threatening condition caused by deposition of proteins that impair kidney function. AL amyloidosis (previously called primary amyloidosis) and AA amyloidosis (previously called secondary amyloidosis) are associated with multiple myeloma (MM) in which kappa or lambda light chains are deposited in the kidney. In the AA type, serum amyloid A (SAA) is an acute-phase reactant deposited in systemic inflammatory disorders such as RA, SLE, CD, or malignancy. These protein deposits damage the glomerular vascular endothelium, allowing protein to enter the urine.

Clinical Presentation. Most cases of amyloidosis affect the kidney, causing nephrotic syndrome and renal failure with foamy urine and edema. The heart (cardiomyopathy, arrhythmia), liver/spleen (hepatosplenomegaly), and tongue (macroglossia) can also be sites of amyloid deposition. In a minority of patients, amyloid fibrils bind to factor X, causing a bleeding diathesis.

Diagnostic Studies.
- Nephrotic-range proteinuria (>3.5 g/day)
- Elevated BUN/creatinine, liver enzymes, and troponins
- Prolonged PT, PTT with low factor X activity
- Serum/urine protein electrophoresis: monoclonal gammopathy suggests MM
- Biopsy of colonic mucosa, gingiva, or abdominal fat pad can confirm amyloidosis

Morphologic Features.
- Microscopic: homogeneous smooth pink extracellular deposits (hyaline material). Congo red stain reveals **"apple green" birefringence** under polarized light
- Electron microscopy: fibrillar deposits

Differential Diagnosis. In a middle-aged patient with new onset kidney disease, diabetes mellitus should be ruled out (hemoglobin A1C $\geq$ 6.5% or fasting glucose $\geq$126 mg/dL is diagnostic of diabetes). Heart failure can cause bilateral lower extremity edema and can be diagnosed with an echocardiogram documenting reduced ejection fraction (EF).

Treatment and Outcomes.

- Patients with amyloidosis are usually evaluated for autologous stem cell transplant; if ineligible, chemotherapy and steroids are usually initiated.
- Patients with multi-organ involvement have a worse prognosis than those with renal-limited disease.

Physiology Correlation. The glomerular filtration apparatus has 3 layers that work together for appropriate filtration of the urine. The capillary endothelial wall has fenestrations (holes) which prevent filtration of blood cells. The next layer, the glomerular basement membrane, is negatively charged and repels negatively charged proteins. Finally, epithelial podocytes have interdigitating slit diaphragms that prevent passage of large molecules such as proteins.

Pharmacology Correlation. Furosemide, a loop diuretic, is often employed to eliminate excess fluid in patients who are volume overloaded. Loop diuretics inhibit a $Na^+/K^+/2Cl^-$ symporter on the luminal membrane of ascending tubules in the loop of Henle. Higher concentrations of these electrolytes in the lumen draw more water into the lumen, resulting in diuresis. Furosemide is a sulfonamide drug that should be avoided in patients with sulfa allergies. Ethacrynic acid, a non-sulfa loop diuretic, notably causes ototoxicity.

Renal and Urinary

Vignette 6

A 32-year-old woman presents to an urgent care clinic complaining of back pain and a low-grade fever of 1-week duration. She has a history of heavy menstrual bleeding with painful cramping but is otherwise healthy. Physical examination is significant for temperature 38.1 C (100.6 F) and an irregular firm, nontender lower abdominal mass. Urine pregnancy test is negative, but urine dipstick is positive for white blood cells and leukocyte esterase.

Pathogenesis. **Chronic obstructive pyelonephritis** develops in patients with long-standing obstruction anywhere between the renal pelvis and urethra, which causes urinary stasis. Any time there is stasis of the urine, there is increased risk of infection, which can cause acute or chronic pyelonephritis. A large nephrolith that fills the renal pelvis can cause unilateral blockage of flow of urine. Prostatic hypertrophy can compress the urethra, while gyneco-logical tumors (uterine fibroids, ovarian cysts or masses) can externally compress one or both ureters. With long-standing obstruction and urinary stasis, the renal pelvis dilates leading to hydronephrosis.

Clinical Presentation. Clinical presentation varies depending on the etiology of the obstruction. With compression of the urethra or external compression of the ureters, patients may be asymptomatic for the obstruction itself and instead present with symptoms related to prostatic hypertrophy (nocturia, hesitancy) or uterine fibroids (painful menstrual cramps and menorrhagia like the patient above). Obstruction by nephroliths can lead to gross hema-turia as the urothelium is damaged by the stone(s); passage of smaller stones through the urethra leads to exquisite colicky abdominal pain.

Diagnostic Studies.
- CBC demonstrates mildly elevated white blood count
- Urinalysis reveals WBCs; depending on etiology, RBCs may be present, too.
- Urine culture and antibiotic susceptibility testing
- U/S of kidneys to visualize hydronephrosis and nephrolithiasis, if present
- BUN and creatinine may be elevated if there is long-standing obstruction affecting both kidneys (as in benign prostatic hyperplasia)

Renal and Urinary

Morphologic Features.

- Gross examination: scars on cortical surface, enlarged **blunted renal calices**
- Microscopic: dilated renal tubules filled with pink colloid-like material (**"thyroidization" of the kidney**), lymphocytes, interstitial fibrosis

Differential Diagnosis. Chronic glomerulonephritis can also cause scarring of the renal cortical surface; however, dilation of the renal pelvis will not be seen. Acute pyelonephritis usually presents with flank pain. *E. coli* is the most common pathogen, due to entry of the bacteria that normally colonize the genital region. Acute cystitis may also be present with suprapubic tenderness.

Treatment and Outcomes.

- Correction of the underlying obstruction may include treating benign prostatic hypertrophy, considering myomectomy for uterine fibroids or lithotripsy for a large kidney stone.
- Empiric antibiotic therapy (ciprofloxacin, ceftriaxone, or piperacillin-tazobactam) can be initiated while awaiting susceptibility testing results.
- If pyelonephritis is left untreated, urosepsis can develop.

Physiology Correlation. Renal clearance is the volume of plasma from which a substance is removed per unit time. To calculate clearance, both the urine concentration, U[X], and plasma concentration, P[X], of the substance and flow rate of urine (V; mL/min) must be known.

$$\text{Clearance (substance X)} = U[X] \times V / P[X]$$

(A mnemonic that might help: clearance = **U V**omit over **P**orcelain).

Pharmacology Correlation. In patients with nephrolithiasis, medical therapy should be initiated to prevent recurrence. Thiazide diuretics increase reabsorption of calcium in the distal convoluted tubule, which decreases calcium content of the urine, reducing the likelihood of precipitation of calcium into stones. Adequate hydration is another mainstay of preventive therapy because it dilutes the urine, making precipitation of stones less likely.

Vignette 7

A 39-year-old man is hired to help clean an old factory that used to manufacture industrial solvents. A coworker accidentally kicks over an unlabeled canister, spilling the sweet-smelling liquid contents. The man starts coughing within 30 minutes and develops a fever 2 hours later, prompting him to go to the ED. The next day, his urine output has decreased and the urine appears dark.

Pathogenesis. **Nephrotoxic acute tubular injury** (or acute renal failure or acute tubular necrosis) can be caused by many things: ischemia from profound hypotension or exposure to nephrotoxic substances (CT contrast media, ethylene glycol, pesticides, carbon tetrachloride, chloroform, myoglobin). These can all lead to potentially-reversible necrosis of the renal tubules.

Clinical Presentation. After exposure to an organic solvent such as carbon tetrachloride, patients usually develop respiratory symptoms such as cough and dyspnea nearly immediately. Within 1-2 days, the patient's urine output decreases (oliguria) or disappears entirely (anuria).

Diagnostic Studies.
- Urine microscopy: **granular/muddy brown casts** from sloughing tubular epithelial cells
- Elevated BUN/creatinine and fractional excretion of sodium (FENa)
- Blood gas shows metabolic acidosis

Morphologic Features.
- Microscopic: coagulative necrosis of renal tubules (loss of nuclei with intensely pink ghost cell outlines), sloughed tubular epithelial cells may be visible in tubular lumens

Differential Diagnosis. Timing and history are key to making the diagnosis. Overdose of NSAIDs—either intentional or unintentional—could also cause nephrotoxic acute tubular injury. Patients with ischemic acute tubular injury typically have signs and symptoms of shock, notably hypotension that leads to inadequate perfusion of the kidneys. Hemolytic uremic syndrome could be another cause of acute kidney injury in a young adult, but there is usually antecedent bloody diarrhea.

Treatment and Outcomes.
- If the inciting nephrotoxic agent is removed, the kidneys have an excellent chance of recovery.
- Patients with poor baseline renal function have a higher risk of progression to chronic kidney injury, necessitating dialysis

Renal and Urinary

Physiology Correlation. FENa is calculated to help determine the etiology of a patient's renal injury. To calculate FENa, the urine and serum concentrations of both sodium and creatinine are needed:

$$\text{FENa (\%)} = \frac{UNa * SCr}{UCr * SNa} * 100$$

- FENa <1% indicates a pre-renal etiology such as hypoperfusion due to hypotension
- FENa >2% indicates an intra-renal etiology such as acute tubular injury
- FENa between 1–2% indicates either a pre-renal or intra-renal cause

Pharmacology Correlation. Activated charcoal (AC) can be employed to prevent toxicity in patients who have overdosed on NSAIDs and orally-ingested poisons. AC binds the toxic substance in the gastric or intestinal lumen, preventing absorption and allowing excretion in the stool. AC is most effective when administered very quickly after ingestion, at most 2 hours later, but ideally within 30 minutes. Vomiting and discoloration of the mouth and fecal material are common side effects.

Vignette 8

A 22-year-old student presents to the health clinic complaining of headaches. She attributed them to stress from studying but they have persisted for several months. Physical examination reveals blood pressure 165/95 mm Hg. She denies smoking. She eats a vegetarian diet and exercises 4 days per week.

Pathogenesis. Fibromuscular dysplasia is caused by hyperplasia of one or more layers of an artery; renal arteries are most commonly involved, but carotid, vertebral, celiac, and mesenteric arteries may also be involved. As layers of the renal artery become thickened, the lumen of the artery becomes focally stenotic with intervening aneurysmal dilation. Over time, this leads to reduced blood flow to the kidney with resultant secondary hypertension (so-called "renovascular hypertension").

Clinical Presentation. Fibromuscular dysplasia is often diagnosed age 20–40, almost exclusively in women. Patients present with headaches due to hypertension, with persistently elevated BP. Flank pain may develop acutely if an aneurysm ruptures or if the affected kidney becomes ischemic. Rarely, an abdominal bruit can be heard on physical examination due to high blood flow through the stenotic renal artery.

Diagnostic Studies.
- **Elevated blood renin level**
- BUN and creatinine are usually normal
- Renal artery **angiography shows "string of beads"** pattern due to irregular stenosis and aneurysm formation
- Excision or biopsy of stenotic artery is almost never performed in contemporary clinical practice

Morphologic Features.
- Multifocal and bilateral (60%) stenoses of the renal arteries
- Microscopy: proliferation of the vascular media layer with narrow/ stenotic lumen

Differential Diagnosis. In the general population, renal artery stenosis is much more commonly caused by atherosclerotic plaques than fibromuscular dysplasia. Coexisting hyperlipidemia is usually identified in patients with atherosclerosis, and patients often have significant risk factors including smoking or diabetes mellitus. Elevated BUN and creatinine are also often seen in atherosclerotic renal artery sclerosis due to plaque rupture causing cholesterol embolization to the renal parenchyma with subsequent ischemia and scarring. Atherosclerosis is very rarely advanced enough in young women to cause stenosis.

Treatment and Outcomes.

- Angiotensin-converting enzyme (ACE) inhibitors (first-line treatment) +/− other antihypertensives
- For those with hypertension refractory to antihypertensives or with bilateral renal artery fibromuscular dysplasia, consider surgical revascularization
- Prognosis depends on maintenance of normal BP: if hypertension remains uncontrolled, patients are at risk for atherosclerosis, coronary artery disease, and stroke

Physiology Correlation. Glomeruli are intimately involved with the regulation of BP by the renin-angiotensin-aldosterone system. Low blood flow is sensed by juxtaglomerular cells in the glomerular afferent arteriole and secrete renin in response. Renin converts angiotensinogen into angiotensin-I, which is subsequently converted to angiotensin-II by ACE. Increased angiotensin-II causes vasoconstriction, which directly increases BP. It also stimulates the adrenal zona glomerulosa to secrete aldosterone, which leads to reabsorption of Na^+ and water to increase plasma volume and thus BP.

Pharmacology Correlation. ACE-inhibitors (lisinopril, enalapril, other *-prils*) prevent the formation of angiotensin II. This prevents vasoconstriction, which in turn reduces BP. One unpleasant side effect of ACE-inhibitors is a chronic dry cough due to buildup of bradykinin; if patients choose to discontinue therapy as a result, angiotensin receptor blockers (ARBs) are an acceptable alternative. ACE-inhibitors should be used with caution or avoided in patients with compromised renal function, as the decrease in renal artery blood flow can cause hypoperfusion and worsening of renal function.

Renal and Urinary

Vignette 9

A 27-year-old man presents to the ED with acute onset flank pain and blood in his urine. Physical examination reveals no abdominal or genital abnormalities. Exam reveals multiple oval-shaped pale macules on his trunk, multiple erythematous papules on his cheeks, and smooth, firm nodules protruding from multiple fingernail beds.

Pathogenesis. **Renal angiomyolipoma** (sometimes called *"AML"* and not to be confused with acute myeloid leukemia) is a type of perivascular epithelioid cell tumor, or PEComa. Renal AMLs develop in a majority of patients with tuberous sclerosis (TS); however, approximately 50% of AMLs develop in patients without TS. TS is caused by an autosomal dominant mutation in tumor suppressor gene *TSC1* (encodes hamartin protein) or *TSC2* (encodes tuberin protein), that stimulates cell growth through the mTOR pathway. This results in the development of hamartomas and other characteristic benign tumors which develop throughout the body, including the skin (ash-leaf spots, angiofibromas, ungual fibroma), brain (subependymal giant cell tumor [SEGA]), heart (rhabdomyoma), and eyes (retinal hamartoma).

Clinical Presentation. Most patients with AML are asymptomatic. The diagnosis is usually made when patients have abdominal imaging performed for an unrelated reason. Due to the vascular component, AMLs occasionally become hemorrhagic, causing flank pain and hematuria. Multifocal angiomyolipoma is more likely than solitary AML to be associated with TS. Patients with TS nearly always have cutaneous findings like the patient above.

Diagnostic Studies.
- Abdominal imaging (CT or MRI) reveals a heterogeneous kidney-based mass (or masses) with fat and hemorrhage
- Bilateral AMLs are strong predictor of TS
- If no evidence of invasive or metastatic disease, surgical resection can be both a therapeutic and diagnostic maneuver without preprocedural biopsy

Morphologic Features.
- Micro: thick-walled blood vessels (*angio-*), bundles of smooth muscle (*-myo-*), and adipose cells (*-lipoma*)
- Minimal to no nuclear atypia
- Positive staining for HMB45

Differential Diagnosis. Nephrolithiasis can cause acute flank pain with hematuria. On imaging, these patients have one or more stones within the urinary tract and do not have an identifiable mass. Urine microscopy may demonstrate crystals. Other renal tumors, such as renal cell carcinoma, can also become hemorrhagic but demonstrate nuclear atypia without triphasic morphology on biopsy or excision.

Treatment and Outcomes.

- Hemorrhagic AMLs are treated by embolization through the renal artery or partial nephrectomy.
- Asymptomatic patients are often observed without intervention.
- AMLs rarely undergo malignant transformation or metastasis. In the absence of severe hemorrhage, prognosis is excellent.

Physiology Correlation. The difference between hypertrophy, hyperplasia, and hamartoma can be confusing.

- Hypertrophy and hyperplasia are physiologic responses to cellular stress; they may coexist depending on the underlying condition (e.g., the gravid uterus demonstrates both)
  - In hypertrophy, individual cells are enlarged but the total number of cells in the organ is not increased
  - In hyperplasia, there is an increase in number of cells
- Hamartomas are benign tumors composed of cells native to the organ in which they are growing

Pharmacology Correlation. Everolimus can be used to treat tumors in TS that are not amenable to surgical resection. Everolimus acts by directly inhibiting mTOR, which reduces cellular proliferation. This medication can also be used as a chemotherapeutic agent for breast cancer, renal cell carcinoma, and neuroendocrine tumors, or as an immunosuppressant for recipients of kidney or liver transplants.

Renal and Urinary

Vignette 10

A 19-year-old college student travels to Egypt during spring break. On a hot day she swims in a river for several hours. A few weeks after returning home, she notices blood in her urine. She denies any new sexual partners, dysuria, increased urination, or vaginal discharge.

Pathogenesis. **Urinary schistosomiasis** (also called vesicular schistosomiasis or *bilharziasis*) is a parasitic infection of the urinary tract with *Schistosoma haematobium*, a trematode or flatworm. This organism is common in parts of Africa, including Egypt; snails residing in fresh water are the usual hosts. The infective form is the cercariae, which penetrate the skin and migrate through blood vessels into the liver where it matures. Adult male/female pairs of worms then enter bladder veins, laying eggs and causing chronic infection. Adult worms of other *Schistosoma* species, such as *S. mansoni* or *S. japonicum*, may establish residence in intestinal veins, causing chronic rectal infection.

Clinical Presentation. Infection should be suspected in travelers to Africa who swim in fresh water. Initial penetration of the organism into the skin causes localized itching. Within a few days of infection, patients may develop a low-grade fever with generalized itching as the organisms disseminate intravascularly, but these symptoms are usually mild or may be absent entirely. With chronic infection, painless hematuria develops.

Diagnostic Studies.
- Urine dipstick or urinalysis positive for blood
- CBC shows **hypereosinophilia**
- Serologic studies for antibodies to *S. haematobium* in the blood
- Urine microscopy may detect **ova in the urine**
- Cystoscopy can help identify polyps that contain ova

Morphologic Features.
- Microscopy: ovoid eggs with a terminal spike surrounded by dense eosinophilic infiltrate within bladder wall. Overlying urothelium may demonstrate squamous metaplasia

Differential Diagnosis. Urinary tract infection is a common cause of acute onset hematuria in a young woman. Dysuria and increased urinary frequency are typically present as well. Hypereosinophilia can be seen in other parasitic infections, or with type I hypersensitivity reactions such as allergic asthma.

Treatment and Outcomes.

- Treat with praziquantel (see pharmacology correlate below).
- If untreated, **risk of progression to bladder squamous cell carcinoma**. This malignancy is otherwise very rare in this location (urothelial/transitional cell carcinoma is by far the most common bladder malignancy).

Physiology Correlation. Eosinophils, one type of white blood cell, are the primary immune cell involved with elimination of parasites. These cells have bilobed nuclei and heavy red (eosinophilic) cytoplasmic granules that contain major basic protein, a peroxidase, and a mast cell chemotactic factor. Eosinophils bind to cell surface antigens of parasites via IgE (type II hypersensitivity), and subsequently degranulate major basic protein.

Pharmacology Correlation. Praziquantel is used to treat schistosomiasis, other trematodes and cestodes (tapeworms). The medication targets helminthic calcium channels, resulting in influx of calcium into the worms. This causes muscle spasms and death of the worm. As the organisms die, eosinophilia may transiently worsen.

Renal and Urinary

Test What You Have Learned

1. A mass is resected from the right kidney of a 2-year-old girl. Microscopic examination shows a triphasic morphology with glandular epithelium, blastema, and stroma. With which of the following would the mass most likely be associated?

   A. Anti-double stranded DNA

   B. Class III hypersensitivity disorders

   C. Hypereosinophilia

   D. Mutation in tumor suppressor gene

   E. Renin angiotensin aldosterone system

   F. Thrombotic microangiopathy

2. A 32-year-old woman complains to her physician that she is having chronic low-grade fevers and that she is tired all of the time. Physical examination demonstrates swollen joints in her fingers. Proteinuria is present on dipstick. Renal biopsy would most likely show which of the following?

   A. "Apple green" birefringence under polarized light

   B. Coagulative necrosis of renal tubules

   C. Positive staining of tumor cells with HMB-45

   D. Proliferation of vascular media layer with narrow lumen

   E. Subendothelial electron-dense deposits

   F. "Thyroidization" of the kidney

3. A 23-year-old woman undergoes abdominal CT scan following an automobile accident. While no injuries related to her accident are found, the scan reveals multifocal large masses in both kidneys. A repeat physical examination demonstrates multiple oval-shaped pale macules on her trunk and small nodules protruding from the edges of some of her finger-nails. A medication with which of the following mechanisms of action might be most useful?

   A. Increases calcium reabsorption in distal convoluted tubule

   B. Inhibits inosine monophosphate dehydrogenase

   C. Inhibits mTOR

   D. Inhibits NKCC2

   E. Prevents mitotic spindle formation

   F. Reduces production of prostaglandins

4. A 23-year-old woman has a headache so severe that she goes to an ED. She states that she has been having these headaches frequently lately, and that she has been trying to ignore them while studying for her college examinations. Her blood pressure in the emergency room is 175/105 mm Hg. Blood renin level is elevated. On further evaluation, which of the following is most likely to be identified?

   A. Fragmented red blood cells

   B. Fusion of podocyte foot processes

   C. Granular/muddy brown casts

   D. WBCs in urine

   E. "String of beads" pattern on renal artery angiography

   F. Urosepsis

5. Two days after visiting a petting zoo, a 7-year-old girl develops severe abdominal pain. She experiences hematochezia and urinalysis reveals RBCs. Her condition would be most likely be related to which of the following?

   A. E. coli O157:H7

   B. Chronic obstructive pyelonephritis

   C. Hodgkin disease

   D. Renovascular hypertension

   E. Schistosomiasis

   F. Tuberous sclerosis

Answers: 1. (D), 2. (E), 3. (C), 4. (E), 5. (A)

CHAPTER 9

Male Reproductive System

Developmental Disorders

❏ Disorders of Sexual Development

 ° Disorders with XY chromosome constitution: testicular regression syndrome, androgen insensitivity syndromes, 5 alpha-reductase deficiency, pure gonadal dysgenesis, rare cases of mixed gonadal dysgenesis

 ° Disorders with abnormal sex chromosome constitution: Klinefelter syndrome, most cases of mixed gonadal dysgenesis

❏ Epispadias
❏ Hypospadias
❏ Cryptorchidism
❏ Ureteropelvic junction obstruction

Inflammatory Conditions

❏ Peyronie disease
❏ Phimosis

Infections

❏ Balanitis
❏ Orchitis
❏ Acute and chronic epididymitis
❏ Acute and chronic prostatitis

Trauma

❏ Testicular torsion

Vascular Diseases

❏ Varicocele

System-Specific Diseases

❏ Prostatic hyperplasia
❏ Hydrocele

Preneoplastic Conditions

❏ Penile intraepithelial neoplasia
❏ Germ cell neoplasia in situ

Neoplasms

❏ Squamous cell carcinoma of the penis
❏ Adenocarcinoma of the prostate
❏ Germ cell tumors of the testis: seminoma, spermatocytic tumor, embryonal carcinoma, yolk sac tumor, choriocarcinoma, teratoma
❏ Sex-cord stromal tumors of the testis: gonadoblastoma, Leydig cell tumor, Sertoli cell tumor
❏ Testicular lymphoma

Representative Diseases

What follows are clinical vignettes for 10 select diseases within this organ system. First, read the vignette and try to identify the condition. Then, move on to read integrated information on each disease.

Vignette 1

A 52-year-old man seeks medical attention for increased pain and scrotal swelling. He also reports unintentional weight loss. Abdominal CT scan shows a mass in the lower right kidney. Biopsy of the mass shows clear cell renal cell carcinoma (RCC), and further genetic testing shows he has mutation of the *VHL* gene.

Diagnosis? _____

Vignette 2

A 12-year-old boy comes to the ED due to a sudden intense pain in the lower abdomen. Abdominal exam shows moderate pain upon deep palpation of the lower abdomen. The scrotum is enlarged and tender. There is no cremasteric reflex.

Diagnosis? _____

Vignette 3

A 31-year-old man who was recently diagnosed with epididymitis comes back a week later with mild scrotal tenderness and swelling. The pain is dull and pressure-like. Transillumination test shows light shining through the scrotum.

Diagnosis? _____

Vignette 4

A 14-year-old boy goes to the clinic with a complaint of constant abdominal fullness. There is evidence of delayed puberty. X-ray of the pelvis shows calcification of the left gonad. A chromosomal analysis is performed.

Diagnosis? _____

Male Reproductive

Vignette 5

A 51-year-old man comes to the clinic complaining of a red, painful lesion on the "head of his private part." Physical exam shows a 2 cm red, velvety plaque on the glans with signs of erosion.

Diagnosis? _____

Vignette 6

A 9-year-old boy comes to the ED with intense right groin pain limiting his ability to walk. He has had myalgia and "puffy cheeks" for a week. Many of his classmates have recently had a febrile illness. Physical exam shows an enlarged right testicle.

Diagnosis? _____

Vignette 7

A 55-year-old man sees his physician after finding a mass on testicular self-examination.

Diagnosis? _____

Vignette 8

On routine checkup a 62-year-old man complains of lower back pain and difficulty voiding. There is a nodule on digital rectum examination.

Diagnosis? _____

Vignette 9

A 62-year-old man is diagnosed with early stage bladder cancer and undergoes intravesical therapy for treatment. Around the time of his second treatment, he goes to see his physician with complaints of severe pain upon urination but no fever or chills. Urinalysis shows increased RBCs and WBCs but no bacterial growth. Labs show increased PSA values.

Diagnosis? _____

Vignette 10

A 27-year-old man comes to the ED with a sudden onset of right-sided back pain and hematuria. U/S shows dilated kidneys and CT confirms the presence of a 1-cm kidney stone obstructing the ureter.

Diagnosis? _____

Vignette 1

A 52-year-old man seeks medical attention for increased pain and scrotal swelling. He also reports unintentional weight loss. Abdominal CT scan shows a mass in the lower right kidney. Biopsy of the mass shows clear cell renal cell carcinoma (RCC), and further genetic testing shows he has mutation of the *VHL* gene.

Pathogenesis. Varicocele is dilatation of the pampiniform plexus. Defective valves are postulated to cause dilatation of the veins. Unilateral (R > L) is the most common presentation, but unilateral (L > R) varicocele is sometimes a secondary to a retroperitoneal tumor that blocks the venous drainage. It is estimated that 15% of men have a varicocele.

Clinical Presentation. Patients with varicocele usually present with dull ache in the scrotum, especially while standing. Some asymptomatic cases are diagnosed during a fertility workup. Other cases come to attention when a tumor enlarges (vignette 1). There are varying grades of varicocele based on ease of clinical detection; the classic description "bag of worms" is not present in every case.

Diagnostic Studies.
- Some cases are palpable on physical exam; others are not.
- Transillumination test: varicocele does not transilluminate
- Scrotal U/S (Doppler mode to assess retrograde flow)

Morphologic Features.
- Gross examination: testicular atrophy
- Microscopic examination: reduced spermatogenesis and maturation arrest

Differential Diagnosis. Hydrocele presents with scrotal swelling that is usually painless. Hydroceles transilluminate and varicoceles do not.

Treatment and Outcomes.
- Conservative/watchful waiting
- Varicocele embolization or surgical ligation of the vein (to maintain fertility)
- NSAIDs for pain management
- Varicocele may increase risk of infertility

Physiology Correlation. Factors contributing to infertility in individuals with varicocele include increased testicular temperature, a decrease in testicular blood flow due to increased vein pressure, and chronic vasoconstriction. These factors all have an effect on spermatogenesis.

Pharmacology Correlation. Discomfort due to varicocele is usually managed first by nonpharmacologic interventions, e.g. athletic supporter, to avoid long-term use of NSAIDs.

Male Reproductive

Vignette 2

A 12-year-old boy comes to the ED due to a sudden intense pain in the lower abdomen. Abdominal exam shows moderate pain upon deep palpation of the lower abdomen. The scrotum is enlarged and tender. There is no cremasteric reflex.

Pathogenesis. **Testicular torsion** is a twisting of the spermatic cord that can infarct the testes. The gubernaculum usually holds the testes in place; however, when there is a laxity or defect in the attachment, the testes have increased mobility and can twist on itself. This twisting of the spermatic cord causes intense pain and ischemia due to decreased vascular flow.

Clinical Presentation. Peak incidence is in infancy and adolescence. Patients experience a sudden, severe pain in the scrotum associated with nausea and vomiting. Pain is worse while walking and can also radiate into the lower abdomen (vignette 2). The testis is tender and mildy enlarged.

Diagnostic Studies.
- Diagnosis is based on clinical signs and symptoms
- Doppler U/S may show absent blood flow

Morphologic Features.
- Gross examination of infarcted testis: dark discoloration, hemorrhage and necrosis: progressive ischemia and infarction of the testis
- Microscopy: intertubular edema, hemorrhage and necrosis of germ cells

Differential Diagnosis. Epididymitis also presents with acute scrotal pain with swelling, but the cremasteric reflex is present. As the name suggests, there is an infectious etiology.

Treatment and Outcomes.
- Immediate urologic evaluation + surgical or manual detorsion
  - If detorsion is performed within 6 hours, there is no loss of testicular viability
  - If not detorsed in 24 hours, there is a complete loss of viability
- Surgical exploration and fixation of both testes.
- Orchiectomy if the testicle is nonviable

Male Reproductive

Physiology Correlation. The cremasteric reflex may be absent in testicular torsion. This reflex is elicited by stroking of the inner part of the ipsilateral thigh. This action stimulates the sensory aspect of the ilioinguinal nerve, which then stimulates the motor fibers of the genital branch of the genitofemoral nerve. This nerve innervates the cremasteric muscle; contraction causes cephalad retraction of the ipsilateral testis.

Pharmacology Correlation. Pain relief is important to the success of manual detorsion. Pain relief helps relax cremasteric fibers; the objective is to control pain enough to allow manipulation for manual detorsion.

Vignette 3

A 31-year-old man who was recently diagnosed with epididymitis comes back a week later with mild scrotal tenderness and swelling. The pain is dull and pressure-like. Transillumination test shows light shining through the scrotum.

Pathogenesis. **Hydrocele** is an accumulation of serous fluid in the tunica vaginalis that causes scrotal enlargement. Because the tunica vaginalis is comprised of 2 layers, there is a potential space between the layers that can be filled with fluid or blood. A recent scrotal infection such as an epididymitis can cause increased fluid production that accumulates in the tunica vaginalis, causing secondary hydrocele. The fluid accumulation can also be idiopathic, due to an imbalance of fluid secretion and reabsorption.

Clinical Presentation. Hydrocele can occur at any age. Patients usually describe a fullness sensation of the affected enlarged scrotum. It occurs gradually and there usually is not much pain involved; if there is, it is usually a pressure-like, tense sensation due to the fluid accumulation.

Diagnostic Studies.

- Physical exam: scrotal swelling
- Transillumination test: transmits light if the fluid is not turbid due to infection
- U/S: hydrocele is avascular on Doppler evaluation

Morphologic Features.

- If chronic, inflammatory infiltration with fibrosis

Differential Diagnosis. A painless, bulging scrotum can be due to an indirect inguinal hernia, which may require surgical evaluation. The mass would not transmit light.

Treatment and Outcomes.

- Antibiotics for infection if indicated
- Drainage if severe infection
- Nonresolving idiopathic hydroceles are evaluated surgically in the pediatric population.

Male Reproductive

Physiology Correlation. The processus vaginalis (tunica vaginalis) usually closes spontaneously by age 1–2. When it does not close following descent of the testis, inguinal hernia or hydrocele may develop.

Pharmacology Correlation. Filarial hydroceles are common in Africa, Asia, the Pacific, and the Middle East. Microfilaricides (e.g. ivermectin) are not completely efficacious and hydrocelectomy is the mainstay of therapy.

Vignette 4

A 14-year-old boy goes to the clinic with a complaint of constant abdominal fullness. There is evidence of delayed puberty. X-ray of the pelvis shows calcification of the left gonad. A chromosomal analysis is performed.

Pathogenesis. Mixed gonadal dysgenesis (MGD) occurs with a mosaicism of 45,X0 and 46,XY genotypes. Due to subpar production of testosterone or Mullerian inhibiting factor by the testes (in either genotypes), the (default) paramesonephric duct continues to form a uterus and the upper part of the vagina (known as **persistent Mullerian structures**). Genital phenotype is ambiguous. Streak gonads, because they are nonfunctioning, have a high likelihood of developing a gonadoblastoma, a tumor with germ cell and stromal elements that has a potential for malignant transformation.

Clinical Presentation. Ambiguous genitalia may be noted in the newborn. Adolescents with MGD have short stature and ambiguous genitalia, and possibly an undescended testis on one side and a streak ovary on the other. There can be partial virilization. Patients who are female phenotypically may seek medical opinion due to amenorrhea. Gonadoblastoma can cause abdominal fullness and pain (vignette 4).

Diagnostic Studies.
- Karyotype
- Retrograde genitography to assess urogenital anatomy
- Gonadal calcification on pelvic x-ray
- CT/MRI of the pelvis
- Testicular biopsy to evaluate for malignancy

Morphologic Features.
- Microscopy of gonadoblastoma: focal calcification comprised mostly with germ cells and Sertoli-like cells in a palisading (enveloping) arrangement around eosinophilic material; cells have small dark nuclei with many mitotic figures

Differential Diagnosis. Turner syndrome also presents with primary amenorrhea in females. The genotype is XO, and affected individuals also have classic phenotypic features such as short stature, wide chest, and webbed neck. Cardiac problems such as bicuspid valve and coarctation of aorta may arise.

Treatment and Outcomes.
- Gonadectomy
- Estrogen / progesterone replacement
- Sex assignment and counseling
- Gonadoblastoma has a high cure rate

Physiology Correlation. Mullerian inhibiting factor is a glycoprotein produced by Sertoli cells that is important in sex differentiation. It causes regression of Mullerian ducts.

Pharmacology Correlation. Estrogen increases osteoclast apoptosis, decreasing the rate of bone resorption. To prevent osteoporosis for those with streak ovaries, estrogen replacement is a consideration.

Vignette 5

A 51-year-old man comes to the clinic complaining of a red, painful lesion on the "head of his private part." Physical exam shows a 2 cm red, velvety plaque on the glans with signs of erosion.

Pathogenesis. Penile intraepithelial neoplasia (PeIN) is a precursor lesion to penile squamous cell carcinomas. Basaloid and warty PeINs are associated with human papilloma virus (HPV), a sexually transmitted infection. **HPV 16** is the most common type associated with these lesions. A non-HPV type of PeIN is called differentiated PeIN. Penile carcinoma is rare in the United States.

Clinical Presentation. Clinical presentation varies. **Erythroplasia of Queyrat** (EQ) (vignette 5) presents on the glans and foreskin and has the highest risk of squamous cancer. Bowen disease occurs as warty lesions on the keratinized shaft of the penis. Small pigmented papules on the shaft of the penis are called *bowenoid papulosis.*

Diagnostic Studies.
- Biopsy of the lesion
- CT or MRI to assess for metastases

Morphologic Features.
- Gross features: The microscopic subtypes cannot be distinguished on gross examination.
- Microscopic examination:
  - Differentiated (HPV-unrelated): acanthosis, parakeratosis, enlarged keratinocytes prominent at bottom layers
  - Basaloid (HPV-related): round basophilic cells with high nuclear/cytoplasmic ratio
  - Warty (HPV-related): bumpy surface (spikes), atypical parakeratosis, and pleomorphic koilocytosis

Differential Diagnosis. Pearly penile papules can look clinically like PeIN but they are not associated with HPV and are not contagious. They typically occur around the corona. Molluscum contagiosum can also occur on the penis; these lesions tend to have an umbilicated center.

Male Reproductive

Treatment and Outcomes.
- Topical 5-fluorouracil (5-FU) cream
- Laser therapy
- Local excision or Moh's micrographic surgery for a penile sparing treatment
- Cryotherapy
- Spread of squamous carcinoma to lymph nodes worsens prognosis, making early detection of PeIN an important clinical goal

Physiology Correlation. Lack of neonatal circumcision and phimosis are risk factors for squamous carcinoma. Lack of circumcision is a factor that is independently associated with detection of HPV in men. Delayed circumcision may not be protective, possibly because inflammatory conditions are already present.

Pharmacology Correlation. 5-fluorouracil is a pyrimidine analog that interferes with DNA synthesis. It is also used to treat skin cancer.

Vignette 6

A 9-year-old boy comes to the ED with intense right groin pain limiting his ability to walk. He has had myalgia and "puffy cheeks" for a week. Many of his classmates have recently had a febrile illness. Physical exam shows an enlarged right testicle.

Pathogenesis. Mumps orchitis is complication that occurs in up to 10% of adolescents and adult men with mumps, an RNA virus of the genus *Paramyxovirus*. Mumps is a highly contagious viral infection that causes systemic inflammation via blood vessels, leading to fever, fatigue, myalgia, and parotitis. The MMR vaccine has reduced the incidence of mumps but outbreaks are still a public health problem. Other complications of mumps include meningitis, encephalitis, mastitis, and oophoritis.

Clinical Presentation. Initially, patients have general malaise with flu-like symptoms such as loss of appetite, fever, fatigue, and myalgia. Parotitis (vignette 6) occurs prior to orchitis. Mumps orchitis usually occurs about 5 days after parotitis. Patients with orchitis experience a sudden onset of fever with severe testicular pain and swelling. Mumps orchitis is unilateral in up to 80% of cases.

Diagnostic Studies.
- Viral diagnosis by serology and culture
- Elevated CRP and amylase
- Blood tests for sexually transmitted infections if indicated
- Doppler U/S showing high blood flow to the testicles

Morphologic Features.
- Testicular atrophy
- Perivascular lymphocytic infiltrate

Differential Diagnosis. Appendicitis can also cause fever and groin pain in addition to pain in the right lower quadrant. McBurney's and Rovsing's signs point toward appendicitis. Testicular torsion is another diagnostic consideration.

Treatment and Outcomes.
- Bed rest, pain medication, and/or ice packs
- Usually resolves in 1 week; potential subfertility

Male Reproductive

Physiology Correlation. Mumps orchitis decreases testosterone levels and increases FSH and LH. In addition to lowering sperm count, orchitis also results in reduced sperm motility (asthenospermia).

Pharmacology Correlation. Over-the-counter painkillers are often used for the pain associated with mumps. To avoid Reye syndrome, children should not take aspirin for relief of mumps symptoms.

Vignette 7

A 55-year-old man sees his physician after finding a mass on testicular self-examination.

Pathogenesis. Spermatocytic tumor is a **germ cell tumor** of the testis. Although once called spermatocytic seminoma, spermatocytic tumor is a separate entity from seminoma, as it differs in histologic, molecular, and clinical features. It is not associated with germ cell neoplasia in situ or cryptorchidism. A gain of chromosome 9 has been reported with these tumors. Personal history of testicular tumor is a risk factor for testicular tumors; a patient with a history of a testicular germ cell tumor has an eight-fold increased risk for a second tumor. Environmental exposure to polyvinyl chlorides, along with history of marijuana and tobacco use, are among some of the risk factors for testicular cancer.

Clinical Presentation. Testicular tumors most often arise in men age <50; however, spermatocytic tumors are less common and usually arise in men age >50. These tumors are quite indolent and can take years for the mass to become noticeable by the patient.

Diagnostic Studies.
- Scrotal U/S
- Serum tumor markers, electrolytes, blood count, liver enzymes and chest x-ray
- CT if seminoma is suspected
- Orchiectomy for definitive tissue diagnosis
- Fine needle biopsy is not optimal for testicular cancers due to the risk of tumor seeding.

Morphologic Features.
- Bilateral tumor in 10%, usually >5 cm at time of diagnosis
- Cut surface is more gelatinous than seminoma
- Microscopy: Sheets and nodules of polygonal cells of varying sizes; giant cells are pleomorphic; mitoses may be numerous; lymphocytes are not a feature
- If sarcomatous (~5% of cases), worse prognosis

Male Reproductive

Differential Diagnosis. Another testicular tumor that can present at age >55 is large B-cell lymphoma. This CD20+ B cell tumor is one of the most common non-Hodgkin lymphomas. Unlike spermatocytic tumor, large B-cell lymphoma is rapidly progressive with a poor prognosis.

Treatment and Outcomes.
- Curative orchiectomy
- Rarely metastasize

Physiology Correlation. Tumor markers are important in the diagnosis and treatment monitoring of testicular cancer. Choriocarcinomas cause elevation of serum hCG, yolk sac tumors cause elevation of AFP; a minority of seminomas cause an elevation of hCG; spermatocytic tumor is not associated with a tumor marker.

Pharmacology Correlation. Because spermatocytic tumors are usually indolent, orchiectomy suffices for treatment and chemotherapy is not part of the treatment.

Vignette 8

On routine checkup a 62-year-old man complains of lower back pain and difficulty voiding. There is a nodule on digital rectum examination.

Pathogenesis. Prostate adenocarcinoma is the most common cancer in men. Risk factors include androgens, family history of prostate cancer (especially in African-Americans), and genetic aberrations (*TMPRSS2-ETS* fusion gene.

Clinical Presentation. Mean age is >65. Patients are usually asymptomatic. When there are symptoms, they are often nonspecific urinary symptoms such as urinary urgency or frequency, which can be experienced with benign prostatic hyperplasia (BPH). Patients may also have a palpable, hard, nodule on digital rectal exam.

Diagnostic Studies.
- Digital rectal exam shows nodular asymmetry
- Serum PSA is elevated (nonspecific for cancer)
- Elevated alk phosphate (if bone metastasis)
- U/S-guided needle biopsy
- X-ray, bone scan, and/or MRI for metastatic lesions

Morphologic Features.
- Gross examination: ill-defined, firm, yellow mass in the peripheral zone of the prostate
- Microscopic features: infiltrating glands with varying arrangements and architectural features, determining Gleason tumor grade

Differential Diagnosis. Benign prostatic hyperplasia (BPH) also presents with urinary symptoms such as frequency and urgency. However, BPH is more likely to cause hematuria and obstructive symptoms such as urinary hesitancy because it tends to occur in the periurethral and transitional zone of the prostate.

Treatment and Outcomes.
- Microscopic tumor grading (Gleason system) for prognosis and therapeutic decisions
- Surgery and radiotherapy if tumor is confined to the prostate
- GnRH-agonist (leuprolide, goserelin) or orchiectomy for metastatic cancers
- Androgen receptor antagonist (flutamide, steroidal cyproterone acetate)

Physiology Correlation. GnRH agonists, when given in pulsatile fashion, stimulate the downstream axis and increase LH/FSH levels. However, continuous administration actually inhibits the axis, decreasing LH/FSH levels, and subsequently inhibits testosterone production.

Pharmacology Correlation. Docetaxel is a chemotherapy used in the treatment of some prostate cancers. It contains ethanol. A known adverse effect is the feeling of intoxication during and after treatment.

Male Reproductive

Vignette 9

A 62-year-old man is diagnosed with early stage bladder cancer and undergoes intravesical therapy for treatment. Around the time of his second treatment, he goes to see his physician with complaints of severe pain upon urination but no fever or chills. Urinalysis shows increased RBCs and WBCs but no bacterial growth. Labs show increased PSA values.

Pathogenesis. BCG prostatitis is an adverse effect of treatment with BCG. BCG therapy is an intravesical immunomodulator that is used to treat bladder cancer. It is derived from a living bovine tubercle bacillus *Mycobacterium bovis*. Because the treatment is intravesical, prostatitis can result as a local complication.

Clinical Presentation. BCG prostatitis causes urinary symptoms of dysuria, urinary urgency and frequency, and sometimes hesitancy and straining.

Diagnostic Studies.
- Urinalysis showing pyuria +/− hematuria
- Urine culture
- U/S, MRI
- PCR for mycobacteria

Morphologic Features.
- Prostate needle biopsy: granulomatous inflammation with caseous necrosis

Differential Diagnosis. Prostatic abscess can also present very similarly to prostatitis. However, imaging would show a distinct pocket of abscess in the prostate.

Treatment and Outcomes.
- Resolves within months of treatment cessation

Physiology Correlation. Prostate-specific antigen (PSA) is a protein that was originally approved by the FDA for treatment monitoring of prostate cancer. It was subsequently approved for prostate cancer screening, but it is not specific for prostate cancer. PSA is also elevated in prostatitis and benign prostatic hyperplasia.

Pharmacology Correlation. In addition to intravesical immunotherapy, intravesical chemotherapy is another treatment option for bladder cancer. Mitomycin is a drug that is administered this way.

Male Reproductive

Vignette 10

A 27-year-old man comes to the ED with a sudden onset of right-sided back pain and hematuria. U/S shows dilated kidneys and CT confirms the presence of a 1-cm kidney stone obstructing the ureter.

Pathogenesis. Ureteropelvic junction (UPJ) obstruction is an impedance of the flow of urine from the kidney to the proximal ureter. Sometimes there is a family history of obstruction. Congenital cases are more common than adult cases. Causes in adults include infection, lithiasis, and iatrogenic injury.

Clinical Presentation. Symptoms include flank pain that occurs on standing or after drinking excessive fluid (Dietl's crisis). Men > women and L > R. Most cases are unilateral.

Diagnostic Studies.
- Increased BUN and Cr
- IVP
- Renal U/S
- CT/MRI
- Prenatal U/S detection (some cases)

Morphologic Features.
- Fibrosis and inflammation due to compression or ischemia
- Abnormal longitudinal muscle bundles and smooth muscle hypotrophy
- Collagen deposition

Differential Diagnosis. Pyelonephritis also can present similarly. Patients with pyelonephritis would most likely also have fever and chills.

Treatment and Outcomes.
- Treat adults based on the underlying etiology (i.e. shock wave lithotripsy for the patient in the vignette)
- Watchful waiting may be appropriate in congenital cases.
- Pyeloplasty may be indicated in some cases.

Physiology Correlation. Congenital UPJ obstruction can occur during development, either via internal stenosis or due to accessory renal artery compression.

Pharmacology Correlation. Thiazide is a commonly used diuretic. It also helps with calcium reabsorption in the distal convoluted tubule, hence this is a treatment of choice for those with calcium oxalate kidney stones (most common) to prevent calciuria. Thiazide is favored for those patients at risk for osteoporosis due to its ability to reabsorb calcium.

Test What You Have Learned

1. A 37-year-old man consults a physician about a 1 cm warty plaque on his penis. Punch biopsy shows atypical parakeratosis and pleomorphic koilocytosis. Which of the following would be most useful in treating this patient medically?

    A. BCG therapy

    B. Finasteride

    C. Leuprolide

    D. NSAIDs

    E. Rifampin

    F. Topical 5-fluorouracil

2. A 42-year-old man consults a physician because his scrotum has been swelling over the last year. The scrotum is mildly tender on examination and transillumination demonstrates light shining through the scrotum. This man's condition is most likely related to which of the following?

    A. Genetic mosaicism

    B. Human papilloma virus infection

    C. Laxity of the gubernaculum

    D. Mumps

    E. Recent scrotal infection

    F. Renal mass

3. A 35-year-old man goes to the emergency room with left-sided back pain. Urinalysis demonstrates blood in the urine. Serum studies show increased BUN and creatinine. CT scan shows dilation of his left ureter. The etiology of this patient's problems would most likely be which of the following?

    A. "Bag of worms"

    B. Enlarged keratinocytes

    C. Granulomatous inflammation

    D. Hemorrhagic infarction

    E. "Streak" gonads

    F. Ureteropelvic junction obstruction

Male Reproductive

4. A 22-year-old man arrives at the ED after a fall while playing football. His scrotum is exquisitely tender. On examination his cremasteric reflex is absent on the right side. Which of the following modalities would best establish the diagnosis?

   A. Core biopsy

   B. CT of pelvis

   C. Doppler U/S

   D. MRI of pelvis

   E. PCR for mycobacteria

   F. Transillumination test

5. A 15-year-old girl is evaluated for failure of menstruation. Ultrasound of the pelvic area demonstrates an undescended testis in the right side of the pelvis and a streak gonad on the left. The streak gonad contains a 2 cm mass. Which of the following additional findings would the patient most likely have?

   A. Endometriosis

   B. High C reactive protein

   C. Hydrocele

   D. Increased white blood cells in urine

   E. Mosaic 45XO and 46XY

   F. Von Hippel-Lindau syndrome

CHAPTER 10
Breast and Female Reproductive System

Checklist of Processes Within This System

Developmental Disorders

❏ Disorders of sexual development: disorders
   with XX chromosome constitution
   (adrenogenital syndrome); disorders
   with other sex chromosome constitution
   (Turner syndrome)
❏ Uterus didelphys
❏ Supernumerary nipple

Infection

❏ Vaginitis
❏ Vaginosis
❏ Pelvic inflammatory disease
❏ Cervicitis
❏ Endometritis
❏ Salpingitis

Trauma

❏ Fat necrosis of the breast
❏ Blunt trauma in pregnancy

System-Specific Processes

❏ Disorders of pregnancy and the
   puerperium: lactating adenoma; mastitis;
   preeclampsia/eclampsia; gestational
   trophoblastic disease; ectopic pregnancy
❏ Squamous intraepithelial lesions: LGSIL
   and HGSIL of the vulva, vagina, and cervix
❏ Nonneoplastic conditions of the
   vulva: lichen sclerosus, lichen simplex
   chronicus, Behçet syndrome, leukoplakia
❏ Polycystic ovary syndrome

❏ Nonneoplastic uterine conditions
   ○ Endometrial hyperplasia
   ○ Endometrial polyps
   ○ Endometriosis
   ○ Adenomyosis

Neoplasia

❏ Stromal tumors of the breast: phyllodes
   tumor; fibroadenoma; sarcoma
❏ Epithelial tumors of the breast and their
   precursors
   ○ Lobular: hyperplasia, lobular carcinoma
     in situ and invasive lobular carcinoma
   ○ Ductal: intraepithelial proliferations,
     ductal carcinoma in situ, invasive duc-
     tal carcinoma (new WHO designation
     "breast carcinoma of no special type")
   ○ special subtypes of invasive breast car-
     cinoma: tubular, cribriform, mucinous,
     and medullary
❏ Squamous carcinoma of the vulva, vagina
   and cervix
❏ Uterine neoplasia
   ○ Endometrial carcinoma
   ○ Uterine leiomyoma
❏ Ovarian tumors
   ○ Epithelial tumors: serous, mucinous,
     endometrioid, Brenner
   ○ Germ cell tumors: dysgerminoma,
     choriocarcinoma, teratoma
   ○ Sex cord-stromal tumors: fibroma, the-
     coma, Leydig cell, granulosa cell, Sertoli

Representative Diseases

What follows are clinical vignettes for 10 select diseases within this organ system. First, read the vignette and try to identify the condition. Then, move on to read integrated information on each disease.

Vignette 1

During a routine checkup, the parents of a 9-year-old girl report that their daughter's classmates call her nicknames pertaining to her short stature. The pediatrician notices the parents are both of average height and that the girl's growth chart reflects slowing of growth rate. The girl is below the 5th percentile for height. The parents deny changes in her diet and appetite. Physical exam is normal. The pediatrician orders labs including a karyotype.

Diagnosis? _____

Vignette 2

A 35-year-old Turkish woman presents with painful ulcers on the vulva and tongue. Physical exam reveals a nodular rash on the legs. A genital swab test is negative. The patient is referred to a dermatologist, who performs a skin prick test which is positive.

Diagnosis? _____

Vignette 3

A 55-year-old woman with complaints of postmenopausal bleeding undergoes vaginal ultrasound. The endometrial lining is found to be diffusely thickened (>4 mm) and an endometrial biopsy is performed. Based on the biopsy results, a course of pharmacologic therapy is recommended.

Diagnosis? _____

Vignette 4

A 64-year-old postmenopausal woman presents with acute left flank pain. She previously had a hysterectomy for fibroids. On exam the abdomen is soft with no palpable mass. Transabdominal sonography reveals left-sided hydronephrosis. On CT there is a space-occupying mass in the ureter, which is resected.

Diagnosis? _____

Vignette 5

A 65-year-old woman presents with complaints of abdominal bloating and distended abdomen. U/S examination reveals ascites. CT exam reveals a 6.0 x 4.8 cm left ovary with a cystic component and omental nodularity.

Diagnosis? _____

Vignette 6

A 41-year-old G0P0 woman with normal BMI and a history of Hashimoto thyroiditis seeks evaluation for infertility. She has taken oral contraceptives for over a decade. Her FSH is within normal limits. Her fertility doctor tells her that her elevated anti-Müllerian hormone indicates she has good ovarian reserve. He does a vaginal U/S, renders his opinion, and suggests medical therapy.

Diagnosis? _____

Vignette 7

A G0P0 45-year-old woman who had tested positive for pregnancy with a commercially available test is told during her first obstetrical visit that a fetus is not identified on U/S. She is told that a D&C and additional lab studies would need to be scheduled for the following day.

Diagnosis? _____

Vignette 8

A 40-year-old G1P0 woman sees the obstetrician for her 36-week appointment. Based on her vital signs and the presence of pedal edema on examination, the physician orders labs. After explaining the results of the lab tests, the obstetrician admits her to the hospital and makes plans for a 37-week induction.

Diagnosis? _____

Vignette 9

A 60-year-old woman undergoes a screening mammography. A small, spiculated mass with a radiolucent core is detected. A stereotactic core needle biopsy is then done, and the histologic diagnosis is radial scar. An excisional biopsy is performed to rule out invasive carcinoma.

Diagnosis? _____

Vignette 10

A 32-year-old woman presents with complaints of a left breast mass. She stopped nursing her newborn 2 weeks ago due to intolerable nipple pain. She is concerned about cancer because her maternal grandmother had breast cancer. On physical exam erythema and induration are noted in the upper inner quadrant of her left breast.

Diagnosis? _____

Vignette 1

> During a routine checkup, the parents of a 9-year-old girl report that their daughter's classmates call her nicknames pertaining to her short stature. The pediatrician notices the parents are both of average height and that the girl's growth chart reflects slowing of growth rate. The girl is below the 5th percentile for height. The parents deny changes in her diet and appetite. Physical exam is normal. The pediatrician orders labs including a karyotype.

Pathogenesis. Turner syndrome (TS) is a common genetic condition occurring in 1 in 2,500 female live births and an unknown number of miscarriages and stillbirths. The chromosomal abnormality is partial or complete loss of the second X chromosome. Half of affected individuals have monosomy X; others have a duplication of the long arm of the X chromosome or mosaicism. Loss of one copy of the *SHOX* gene affects growth and bone development.

Clinical Presentation. Diagnosis occurs at different stages of life because phenotypic features may be subtle or lacking. Prenatal U/S findings may include increased nuchal translucency, cystic hygroma, and renal and/or left-sided cardiac anomalies. In infancy there may be redundant nuchal skin, lymphedema of the hands and feet, and congenital heart defects; infants with 45,X karyotype are more likely to have lymphedema. In childhood, when about a third of cases are diagnosed, signs may include delayed puberty and short stature, which is the most common finding and the presenting sign in vignette 1. Some cases may not be recognized until loss of ovarian function is detected during infertility workup.

Diagnostic Studies.

- During pregnancy: abnormal maternal quadruple serum screening test necessitates amniocentesis or chorionic villus sampling for fetal karyotyping for definitive diagnosis
- When karyotyping blood samples, >20 cells may need to be counted to detect some cases of mosaicism
- In individuals with known TS, routine examinations are important; for example, echocardiography is done at regular intervals to screen for aortic root dilatation

Morphologic Features.

- Streak ovaries
  - Macroscopic: a streak of fibrous tissue in the usual ovarian location.
  - Microscopic: normal ovarian cortex without germ cells.
- Gonadoblastoma (present in some TS patients):
  - Macroscopic: smooth outer surface with a granular cut surface.
  - Microscopic: germ cells and immature sex-cord stromal cells, calcification; dysgerminoma may also be present.

Differential Diagnosis. In children presenting with facial dysmorphology, webbed neck, and congenital heart defects, the differential diagnosis includes Noonan syndrome, an autosomal dominant condition caused by gene mutations that alter the Ras/MAPK cell signaling pathway. The karyotype is normal in Noonan syndrome and diagnosis is based on clinical features.

Treatment and Outcomes.

- Growth hormone (GH) to optimize final adult height.
- Oxandrolone (an anabolic steroid) if GH alone does not significantly increase height.
- Hormone-replacement therapy with transdermal 17-β estradiol (TDE) and progestin to achieve normal development and optimal bone mass.
- Some affected fetuses spontaneously abort.
- There is usually normal intelligence although varying degrees of neuro-cognitive and psychosocial challenges may develop.
- Cardiovascular abnormalities can shorten lifespan.
- Endocrine disorders (e.g., hypothyroidism in individuals with an iso-chromosome Xq) and infertility are common.
- In girls with mosaicism for a population with a Y chromosome, a gonadoblastoma may develop in a streak ovary.

Physiology Correlation. Growth hormone is secreted by somatotropes in the anterior pituitary under the control of somatotropin-releasing hormone and somatostatin. GH has an anabolic function. Its effect on skeletal growth is mediated by polypeptides called somatomedins, which are produced in the liver and bone. Hyposecretion of GH causes dwarfism, and hypersecretion causes gigantism in children and acromegaly in adults. GH is secreted in hypoglycemia; although it has an antiinsulin effect, the somatomedins have insulin-like effects.

Pharmacology Correlation. Sourcing GH from cadaveric pituitaries was discontinued in the 1980s due to reports of Creutzfeldt-Jakob disease; recombinant GH is now used as replacement therapy. Treatment with GH begins as early as age 4–6 years to increase adult height; studies have reported a gain in adult height of 5–8 cm. Outcomes depend on factors including patient age at the start of treatment and duration of treatment. The hormone is administered subcutaneously at night when it is normally released from the pituitary. Dose is calculated from patient weight in kilograms. Treatment may worsen an already increased risk of insulin resistance; the dose is adjusted based on concentrations of IGF-I (insulin-like growth factor I), which are periodically monitored.

Vignette 2

A 35-year-old Turkish woman presents with painful ulcers on the vulva and tongue. Physical exam reveals a nodular rash on the legs. A genital swab test is negative. The patient is referred to a dermatologist, who performs a skin prick test which is positive.

Pathogenesis. **Behçet Disease** (BD) is a rare inflammatory disorder of unknown cause that occurs most often in men and women with Middle Eastern and Asian heritage.

Clinical Presentation. Manifestations of relapsing and remitting multiorgan involvement are characteristic; mucocutaneous lesions, ocular findings, and a rash are classic but are not always present at the same time; for example, **oral aphthosis** may precede genital ulcerations by years. In men genital ulcers typically occur on the scrotum, while in women they occur on the vulva. Eye involvement may occur early or late, causing photophobia, pain, tearing, and even blindness. Other manifestations involve the skin (eruptions) vessels (thrombophlebitis), CNS (headache, stroke and seizures) and GI tract (diarrhea and bleeding).

Diagnostic Studies.

- No gold standard test; multiple versions of diagnostic criteria have been proposed
- One internationally recognized set of criteria assigns a varying number of points to pertinent clinical findings such as ocular lesions or CNS involvement
- Totality of the clinical findings, as established by multiple specialists, is key to diagnosis
  - An ophthalmologist will perform a fundic exam to look for uveitis
  - A dermatologist will perform a **pathergy test** (skin prick test); the positive pathergy reaction seen in BD is similar to the Koebner phenomenon of psoriasis
- HLA testing may support a diagnosis; BD is more common in HLA-B51+ and HLA-B5+ individuals

Differential Diagnosis. Reactive arthritis is an inflammatory disorder presenting with multiorgan involvement after an extraarticular infection, but patients are more often HLA B27+. Stevens-Johnson syndrome also causes bullous lesions on the mouth and genitals; skin biopsy shows full thickness epidermal necrosis with minimal inflammation. Sweet syndrome causes fever, arthritis and rash, often after a short flulike illness; neutrophils are noted in the dermis on biopsy.

Morphologic Features.
- Vulva biopsy: a neutrophilic response in the ulcer center with a lymphocytic response at the periphery.
- Skin biopsy of a papulonodular lesion: lymphocytic dermal infiltrate.

Treatment and Outcomes.
- There is no curative therapy.
- NSAIDs for BD-related arthritis
- Colchicine for joint symptoms and erythema nodosum
- Azathioprine and cyclosporine A for ocular disease
- Thalidomide for orogenital ulcerations
- Remission and relapse are common.
- In about 30% of cases, thrombosis may lead to morbidity and mortality.

Physiology Correlation. BD predisposes to venous and arterial thrombosis. Superficial and deep thrombophlebitis, thrombosis of the vena cava, and intracardiac thrombus have all been reported with BD. Thrombosis is the formation of clot inside a blood vessel. In general, 3 factors which predispose to thrombosis are hemodynamic factors, vascular factors, and blood factors. Increases in von Willebrand factor have been reported in individuals with BD, and inflammatory changes are often present in vessel walls. Anticoagulant therapy has not consistently prevented recurrence of thrombosis in BD, and it has not been studied in randomized controlled trials.

Pharmacology Correlation. Topical steroid cream is used to treat the genital ulcers of BD. Topical steroids are available in 7 groups of potency. Epidermal atrophy can develop depending on the length of use, potency and age of the patient, with extremes of age being more susceptible to the side effect. Topical steroids are absorbed through intact skin; if the skin is inflamed or covered with an occlusive bandage, absorption may be increased. Systemic absorption of topical steroids can cause suppression of the hypothalamic-pituitary-adrenal axis. Metabolism occurs primarily in the liver with excretion in the kidney.

Vignette 3

A 55-year-old woman with complaints of postmenopausal bleeding undergoes vaginal ultrasound. The endometrial lining is found to be diffusely thickened (>4 mm) and an endometrial biopsy is performed. Based on the biopsy results, a course of pharmacologic therapy is recommended.

Pathogenesis. Benign hyperplasia (BH) of the endometrium (formerly known as hyperplasia without atypia) is a proliferation of the endometrial lining that causes uterine bleeding. Over 30% of women experience abnormal uterine bleeding (AUB) in the course of their life: heavy menstrual, irregular/intermenstrual, or postmenopausal bleeding. The postmenopausal endometrium is usually atrophic but can undergo hyperplasia due to unopposed estrogenic stimulation. Etiologic factors causing postmenopausal endometrial stimulation include anovulation, obesity, and metabolic syndrome. Risk is also increased in nulliparous women. Tamoxifen (a breast cancer treatment) and hormone replacement therapy (with unopposed estrogen) increase risk. Genetic alterations that have been identified with hyperplasia include loss of *PTEN* and *PAX2*. At the molecular level, hyperplasia results from disruption/inhibition of apoptosis in endometrial cells. Endometrial hyperplasia is a precursor to type I endometrial carcinoma. Risk of carcinoma is lower in hyperplasia without atypia, called benign hyperplasia, than it is in hyperplasia with atypia, now called endometrial intraepithelial neoplasia (formerly known as hyperplasia with atypia).

Clinical Presentation. Mean age is 52. Symptoms include heavy uterine bleeding (menorrhagia), intermenstrual bleeding (metrorrhagia) and postmenopausal bleeding.

Diagnostic Studies.

- Transvaginal ultrasonography to evaluate the thickness of the endometrium; endometrial thickness <4 mm has negative predictive value for carcinoma in 99% of cases
- Hysteroscopy to noninvasively visually inspect the endometrial surface; often done when a biopsy returns with a diagnosis of atypical hyperplasia
- Endometrial biopsy/curettage to determine if premalignant or malignant process is present, especially in women with risk factors for endometrial carcinoma

Differential Diagnosis. The International Federation of Gynecology and Obstetrics (FIGO) uses the PALM-COEIN acronym to identify the differential of AUB. PALM-COEIN is **p**olyp, **a**denomyosis, **l**eiomyoma, **m**alignancy/hyperplasia, **c**oagulopathy, **o**vulatory dysfunction, **e**ndometrial, **i**atrogenic, and **n**ot otherwise classified. Age is an important consideration. In prepubertal girls, the lower genital tract (not the uterus) is often the source of bleeding, and the differential includes trauma, foreign body and vulvovaginitis. In adolescents, anovulatory uterine bleeding is the most common cause of AUB. In the reproductive age group, when AUB most frequently presents, endometrial polyps, leiomyomas, and adenomyosis are the most common cause of AUB.

One pitfall in diagnostic surgical pathology is that an endometrial polyp can be misdiagnosed as endometrial hyperplasia, but it is also true that polyps can contain hyperplastic glands and even adenocarcinoma. Microscopic recognition of a fibrous core with thick-walled vessels is key to diagnosing a polyp in a biopsy specimen. In postmenopausal women, important disease considerations for vaginal bleeding include vaginal atrophy, cervical carcinoma and endometrial carcinoma. Because vaginal bleeding is the presenting symptom of endometrial cancer in >90% of cases, it is important to exclude endometrial carcinoma by histologic examination. Although the wordings are similar, *endometrial intraepithelial neoplasia* and *endometrial intraepithelial carcinoma* are not interchangeable terms; the latter references a precursor to a serous (type II) carcinoma of the endometrium.

Morphologic Features.
- Overall, hyperplasia is an increased volume of endometrial tissue with an increased ratio of glands to stroma.
- Nuclear atypia is used to discern benign hyperplasia (BH) from endometrial intraepithelial neoplasia (EIN); nuclear atypia is present in the latter.

Treatment and Outcomes.
- For benign hyperplasia, progestin administration with follow-up biopsy. If response to therapy occurs, it is usually within 6 months.
- For hyperplasia with atypia, surgical hysterectomy (25–50% of cases progress to carcinoma or present concurrently with carcinoma)

Physiology Correlation. Estrogen causes proliferation of the endometrium; progesterone mitigates the effects of estrogen. After ovulation, progesterone levels rise to prepare the endometrium for potential implantation. Endogenous or exogenous (e.g., hormone replacement therapy) unopposed estrogenic stimulation of the endometrium is a risk factor for carcinoma.

Pharmacology Correlation. Progestin is a synthetic progesterone used for nonsurgical treatment of endometrial hyperplasia. Routes of administration include oral, intramuscular, and implanted intrauterine device. Side effects include headache, cramping, and uterine bleeding. Resistance to therapy can occur due to inadequate or altered receptor function.

Vignette 4

A 64-year-old postmenopausal woman presents with acute left flank pain. She previously had a hysterectomy for fibroids. On exam the abdomen is soft with no palpable mass. Transabdominal sonography reveals left-sided hydronephrosis. On CT there is a space-occupying mass in the ureter, which is resected.

Pathogenesis. **Endometriosis** is an estrogen-dependent disease characterized by the benign, invasive growth of endometrial tissue in ectopic locations. Although it can be present in extraperitoneal locations including the CNS and lungs, involvement is typically in the pelvis in locations such as the ovaries and ligaments. This ectopia is postulated to arise from stem cells, metaplasia, or menstrual backflow through the fallopian tubes. Establishment of the ectopic endometrial tissue relies on neovascularization. COX enzymes and prostaglandins play a role in the pathology, which is now postulated to include immune and hormonal factors.

Endometriosis is a common condition affecting 10% of women during their reproductive years. Risk factors include family history, obesity and unopposed estrogen use. Endometrial tissue, even in an ectopic location, is sensitive to estrogen. Under normal circumstances, during the proliferative phase of the menstrual cycle, estrogen stimulates regeneration of the stratum functionalis and induces mitosis. Endometriotic tissue is under the same hormonal influences and undergoes cyclical changes, including bleeding.

Clinical Presentation. Symptoms may be nonspecific: chronic pelvic pain, dysmenorrhea, and dyspareunia. When endometriosis affects distant sites, the clinical presentation varies with the site of involvement. Abnormal bleeding such as vaginal bleeding, rectal bleeding, hematuria or hemoptysis may be the presenting symptom. While the patient with ureteral involvement of endometriosis in the vignette suffered flank pain, >50% of cases of ureteral endometriosis are in fact asymptomatic; in some cases there is a resulting loss of renal function. Fortunately, ureteral involvement is extremely rare in women with this condition.

Diagnostic Studies.
- Pending the development of biomarkers for diagnosis, laparoscopy is the mainstay for definitive diagnosis
  - Allows visualization and tissue sampling of foci of endo, but typically a course of medical treatment is provided before the invasive test is performed
  - The nonspecific clinical presentation and invasive nature of the definitive diagnostic procedure can delay diagnosis for years
- Transvaginal U/S to identify ovarian endometriomas
- CT and MRI to preoperatively stage endometriosis

Differential Diagnosis. The symptom of pain may elicit an investigation for pelvic inflammatory disease, ovarian torsion, and acute abdomen. A vaginal swab can diagnose infection. Abdominal and pelvic examination along with laboratory studies may help to rule out the other conditions, but they don't provide information to definitively diagnose endometriosis.

Morphologic Features.

- Foci of endometriosis may appear brown and hemorrhagic on the surface of the involved tissue. In the ovary there may be large, fluid-filled brown cysts.
- Microscopic diagnosis requires the finding of endometrial glands or stroma. Incidental microscopic identification of glands with tubal epithelium outside of the fallopian tubes is called endosalpingiosis and is distinct from endometriosis.
- Microscopically, stromal endometriosis (uterine stroma without glands) may be identified in the ovary.
- The endometriotic glands may undergo hyperplastic change. In post-menopausal women the glands are often atrophic.

Treatment and Outcomes.

- There is no cure for endometriosis, and treatment is aimed at alleviating pain or restoring fertility; these aims are in ways at odds with each other.
- Medical therapy to reduce pain does not improve fertility and is actually contraindicated in women trying to conceive.
- Pharmacologic therapy for pain includes combined oral contraceptives, NSAIDs, and gonadotropin-releasing hormone (GnRH) analogs.
- Surgical excision of endometriotic tissue may relieve pain and improve fertility.
- Complications of endometriosis include bleeding, rupture of cysts, and adhesion formation.

Physiology Correlation. The hypothalamus secretes hormones that control visceral functions. GnRH is secreted by the hypothalamus and acts on the pituitary to control the synthesis and secretion of follicle-stimulating hormone (FSH) and luteinizing hormone (LH). The release of GnRH is subject to feedback loops in the hypothalamic-pituitary-gonadal axis.

Pharmacology Correlation. GnRH analogs (also known as luteinizing hormone release agonists) are sometimes used to treat the pain of endometriosis; they reduce estrogen levels. Upon initial administration, they stimulate pituitary gonadotropin release, but over time the stimulation triggers an inhibition of gonadotropin secretion. Leuprolide acetate is injected. Hypoestrogenic side effects include vasomotor symptoms (hot flashes) and a reduction in bone mineral density; therefore, long-term use of the drug is limited. Hormonal add-back therapies with progestins are sometimes used to offset bone mineral loss.

Vignette 5

A 65-year-old woman presents with complaints of abdominal bloating and distended abdomen. U/S examination reveals ascites. CT exam reveals a 6.0 x 4.8 cm left ovary with a cystic component and omental nodularity.

Pathogenesis. **High-grade serous carcinoma (HGSC)** is the most common type of ovarian cancer. Recent research points to the origin of HGSC in intraepithelial carcinomas of the fimbriated end of the fallopian tube. During embryonic development, the fallopian tube arises from the Mullerian duct; the ovaries and urinary tract arise from mesoderm. The historical concept of HGSC arising from Mullerian metaplasia has been cast out in part due to histopathological studies of ovarian cancer resection specimens that identified serous tubal intraepithelial tumors (STICs). This work was further supported by increased p53 signatures in STIC tubes; *TP53* mutation is present in 80% of cases of HGSC. Ten percent of ovarian cancers are caused by BRCA1/2 mutation. Notch signaling is also an important oncogenic pathway. Family history of ovarian cancer in a first-degree relative is the most important known risk factor.

Clinical Presentation. Mean age is 55–65. HGSC presents at advanced stage, as in the vignette where the omental nodularity represented metastases. Symptoms are nonspecific and may include abdominal pain, vaginal discharge and postmenopausal bleeding. Tumors are often bilateral; at time of diagnosis, disease is widespread to lymph nodes and the peritoneum.

Diagnostic Studies.
- Pelvic exam and transvaginal U/S to help reveal a possible mass
- Increased levels of CA-125 are not specific to ovarian carcinoma
- Microscopic examination of surgical pathology specimens is necessary for precise diagnosis.

Morphologic Features.
- Gross examination of the ovaries
  - Massively enlarged ovary; bilateral involvement frequently occurs.
  - The tumor has a cystic or solid cut surface with foci of necrosis and hemorrhage.
- Microscopic examination of the ovarian tumor
  - Sporadic and germline cases are microscopically identical.
  - Variable architecture: large papillae, glandular pattern, solid sheets of tumor cells
  - High grade nuclei with a high mitotic index.

Differential Diagnosis. The distinction between low grade and high grade serous carcinoma is based on nuclear features and is significant given that survival differences are measured in years. Microscopic examination is necessary to distinguish HGSC from other forms of ovarian carcinoma. Other tumors with microscopic papillae include endometrioid carcinoma and clear cell carcinoma.

Treatment and Outcomes.
- Cytoreductive surgery
  - Platinum- and taxane-based chemotherapy
  - Recurrence is common and tumors become refractory to chemotherapy
- Compared to sporadic cases, BRCA1/BRCA2-mutant forms of HGSC have increased long-term survival.
- 5-year survival rate <35%.

Physiology Correlation. CA125 is a serum tumor marker also known as mucin 16. It is transmembrane mucin produced by the epithelium of the eye, GI tract, and gynecologic tract. The gene coding for this protein, *MUC16*, is mutated in tumors including pancreatic and colorectal adenocarcinoma. In the normal physiologic state, levels of this protein fluctuate with the menstrual cycle. In terms of tumor biology, the protein is involved in metastasis and resistance to chemotherapy. While it is not used as a screening test for ovarian cancer (there are still no approved screening tests for ovarian cancer), the serum concentrations of the protein are monitored during ovarian cancer therapy; increased levels correlate with relapse.

Pharmacology Correlation. Carboplatin is an alkylating agent that targets DNA synthesis. HGSC has a better response to taxane-and platinum-based chemotherapy than low grade tumors. Nonetheless, HGSC develops resistance to these agents. Over half of the carboplatin dose is eliminated in urine within 24 hours. Patients with impaired renal function require lower doses because the drug is excreted by glomerular filtration. The drug causes myelosuppression. Renal function and peripheral blood counts are monitored in patients.

Vignette 6

A 41-year-old G0P0 woman with normal BMI and a history of Hashimoto thyroiditis seeks evaluation for infertility. She has taken oral contraceptives for over a decade. Her FSH is within normal limits. Her fertility doctor tells her that her elevated anti-Müllerian hormone indicates she has good ovarian reserve. He does a vaginal U/S, renders his opinion, and suggests medical therapy.

Pathogenesis. Polycystic ovary syndrome (PCOS) is a complex endocrine disease whose precise pathogenesis remains undetermined. Genetic and environmental factors are thought to play a role. Classic features are hyperandrogenism, anovulation, and insulin resistance. Obesity worsens the metabolic derangements and subfertility associated with PCOS.

Clinical Presentation. PCOS affects approximately 10% of reproductive-aged women. There are 2 phenotypes associated with PCOS. The classical one is characterized by truncal obesity, hirsutism, menstrual irregularities, and metabolic syndrome. The lean PCOS phenotype can occur in women with low BMI with few or absent signs of hyperandrogenism. PCOS is the most common cause of female infertility, and in some cases, diagnosis is not made until a woman is evaluated for assisted reproductive technology, as was the case with the woman in the vignette.

Morphologic Features.

- Gross examination of ovaries: ovaries may be enlarged; cysts (arrested antral follicles) (35% of cases) are seen below the surface
- Microscopic examination of ovaries: collagenization of outer ovarian cortex; multiple follicle cysts with luteinized theca cells (corpora lutea and albicantia are typically absent)

Diagnostic Studies.

- Diagnosis is based on a constellation of laboratory findings, plus a complete history and physical exam, including menstrual history, calculation of body mass index, notation of phenotypic features of hyperandrogenism (acne, oily skin, hirsutism), palpation of ovaries
- Antral follicle count may be obtained from U/S
- Serum testosterone and the ratio of LH/FSH may be increased.

Differential Diagnosis.

- In the setting of menstrual irregularities and hyperandrogenism, PCOS is a diagnosis of exclusion and other conditions should be considered in the differential

- In late-onset congenital adrenal hyperplasia, increased ACTH levels cause increased androgen secretion
- Lab analysis to exclude congenital adrenal hyperplasia
- Early Cushing's syndrome is sometimes misdiagnosed as PCOS
- Hypothyroidism, prolactin excess, acromegaly, and androgen secreting tumors are other diagnostic considerations.

Treatment and Outcomes.
- Diet for weight loss to improve hyperandrogenemia and ovulatory function.
- Oral contraceptives to normalize androgen levels.
- Ovulation induction with clomiphene in women seeking fertility assistance.
- Women with hyperandrogenism have a higher incidence of cardiovascular disease, hyperlipidemia, and diabetes.
- There is an increased risk of endometrial carcinoma and gestational diabetes mellitus.

Physiology Correlation. Normally in females, half of testosterone derives from the peripheral conversion of circulating androstenedione (in the liver, skin and fat) and half derives from the ovary and adrenal glands in response to LH and ACTH, respectively. Androgens are not under negative feedback control by pituitary trophic hormones. Insulin excess downregulates intraovarian mechanisms to control androgen production. Androgen excess promotes proliferation of small antral follicles and also negatively impacts follicle maturation. Anti-Müllerian hormone is produced by small antral follicles.

Pharmacology Correlation. Clomiphene citrate induces ovulation by inducing follicle growth; it is a first-line oral therapy for infertility. This selective estrogen receptor modulator has adverse effects including multiple pregnancy, thromboembolism, visual changes (scintillating scotomata), ovarian enlargement, and ovarian hyperstimulation syndrome (ovarian enlargement and third spacing leading to ascites). The drug can cause enlargement of uterine fibroids.

Vignette 7

A G0P0 45-year-old woman who had tested positive for pregnancy with a commercially available test is told during her first obstetrical visit that a fetus is not identified on U/S. She is told that a D&C and additional lab studies would need to be scheduled for the following day.

Pathogenesis. A **hydatidiform mole** (HM) is a placental disease that arises from an abnormal fertilization. The gestational trophoblastic diseases (GTDs) are a group of benign (partial and complete hydatidiform mole) and malignant (gestational trophoblastic neoplasia) disorders of trophoblastic tissue. Hydatidiform mole is the most common type of gestational trophoblastic disease. The incidence of molar pregnancy is 1–3 per 1000 pregnancies; it occurs more often in Asian and Latin American populations and more often at women at the extremes of the reproductive spectrum. A **complete hydatidiform mole** has a diploid karyotype (more often 46,XX) with both X chromosomes of paternal origin, which results from duplication of haploid sperm. A **partial hydatidiform mole** is usually triploid (more often 69,XXY or 69,XXX) with a paternal extra set of chromosomes. Half of all cases of gestational trophoblastic neoplasia occur after a molar pregnancy. Gestational trophoblastic neoplasia includes invasive mole, choriocarcinoma, placental site trophoblastic tumor and epithelioid trophoblastic tumor. Invasive mole is the most common form after molar pregnancy and is more common than choriocarcinoma.

Clinical Presentation. Hydatidiform mole can present with vaginal bleeding; hyperemesis gravidarum is present in some cases. Early preeclampsia is a rare presenting symptom. Uterine size is often large for dates in cases of complete mole; in partial hydatidiform mole, uterine size is often small for dates. As in the vignette, some cases are asymptomatic and are detected in the first trimester by routine obstetric U/S.

Diagnostic Studies.

- Classic finding of complete HM on ultrasonography is "snowstorm" pattern that correlates with the mass of vesicles, but this finding may not be present in the first trimester
- Microscopic examination of evacuated material is necessary to distinguish among the types of GTD
- Serum beta-hCG to diagnose and monitor trophoblastic disease
  - In partial HM, serum hCG is low or normal for gestational age
  - After evacuation of a molar pregnancy, serial serum hCG levels are followed; a plateau or rise in hCG indicates the presence of GTN.
- Chest x-ray to detect pulmonary metastases of GTN

Morphologic Features.
- Gross appearance of evacuated specimen: a mass of cystic vesicles
- Microscopic findings of evacuated specimen
  - Complete mole: villous edema and circumferential trophoblastic proliferation
  - Partial mole: only some villi are edematous and trophoblastic proliferation is focal

Differential Diagnosis. Although the clinical presentation can be helpful, specific diagnosis is made by microscopy. On histologic examination of evacuated tissue, some pregnancies suspected to be HM by ultrasonography instead represent cases of nonmolar hydropic abortions. In some cases where spontaneous abortion is the working clinical diagnosis, HM is diagnosed on the basis of the pathologist's microscopic examination of the curettage specimen.

Treatment and Outcomes.
- For HM, surgical evacuation and monitoring of **serial beta-hCG levels** to screen for gestational trophoblastic neoplasia; contraception is recommended for a year during follow-up of hCG. Invasive mole occurs in about 15% of HM cases.
- GTN may occur years after the diagnosis of HM.
- If gestational trophoblastic neoplasia is diagnosed, division into low-risk and high-risk groups forms the basis for treatment protocols.
- Invasive mole is treated with the low-risk GTN protocol, single-agent chemotherapy. Untreated invasive mole may cause uterine perforation.
- High-risk GTN is treated with polychemotherapy.
- Over 80% of women with GTN are cured.

Physiology Correlation. The trophoblast is the site of placental hormone production. It produces hCG along with other hormones including estrogen and progesterone. Levels of hCG peak by the end of the second trimester before falling to an undetectable level at term.

Pharmacology Correlation. Methotrexate (MTX) is one drug used in single-agent therapy for GTN. It is a competitive inhibitor of dihydrofolate reductase, which is required for DNA and RNA synthesis. MTX selectively acts on rapidly dividing cells, making it useful for treatment of some cancers. Oral mucositis can occur. The drug is excreted in urine, and conditions changing renal function increase risk of toxicity.

Breast and Female Reproductive

Vignette 8

A 40-year-old G1P0 woman sees the obstetrician for her 36-week appointment. Based on her vital signs and the presence of pedal edema on examination, the physician orders labs. After explaining the results of the lab tests, the obstetrician admits her to the hospital and makes plans for a 37-week induction.

Pathogenesis. Preeclampsia is a pregnancy-related hypertension syndrome characterized by the new onset of hypertension and either proteinuria or end-organ dysfunction in a previously normotensive woman. It is caused by altered trophoblastic invasion and remodeling of maternal spiral arteries that leads to placental hypoperfusion. The exact cause of the placental hypoperfusion remains unknown, but resulting placental pathogenic factors enter the maternal circulation and drive the disease process. Risk factors for preeclampsia include maternal chronic kidney disease, maternal hypertension, maternal diabetes type 1 or 2, maternal autoimmune disease (e.g., antiphospholipid syndrome), and previous history or family history of preeclampsia. It is an important cause of maternal and infant mortality, and it occurs in ~5% of pregnancies.

Clinical Presentation. This disease usually presents in the third trimester of pregnancy. Some cases, even severe cases, are asymptomatic. Symptoms of severe preeclampsia may include headaches, epigastric pain, shortness of breath and abdominal pain. Eclampsia is the new onset of a grand mal seizure in a woman diagnosed with preeclampsia.

Diagnostic Studies.

- Diagnosis is based largely on evidence of end-organ injury
- Hypertension is present and proteinuria may or may not be present; other criteria include thrombocytopenia of new onset, altered liver function, renal insufficiency, and cerebral or visual symptoms
- Maternal CBC, liver enzymes and serum creatinine are monitored
- Fetal examination includes a nonstress test (screening test based on fetal heart rate), and biophysical profile (utilizing a fetal U/S that also estimates amniotic fluid levels) if nonstress test is nonreactive

Morphologic Features.

- Gross examination of placenta
  - Relatively small in size
  - More numerous infarcts
  - Retroplacental hematoma in a small percentage of cases

- Microscopic findings in the placenta:
  - Small villi
  - Villous syncytial knots
- Microscopic findings in maternal spiral arteries
  - Acute atherosis (fibrinoid necrosis of vessel wall and accompanying lipid-containing macrophages)

Differential Diagnosis. The differential diagnosis includes other types of hypertension in pregnancy. Chronic hypertension is usually present before 20 weeks gestation, and preeclampsia often does not cause hypertension until after 20 weeks gestation. It is possible for preeclampsia to be superimposed on chronic hypertension. Gestational hypertension (formerly called pregnancy-induced hypertension) occurs after 20 weeks gestation but lacks the other features of preeclampsia. It can be difficult to distinguish preeclampsia from a flare of lupus nephritis because lupus is a risk factor for preeclampsia.

Treatment and Outcomes.

- Hemorrhagic stroke, hemolysis, elevated liver enzymes, and low platelets (HELLP syndrome) may arise as a complication.
- Short-acting parenteral antihypertensive drugs are used in severe cases of preeclampsia.
- Magnesium sulfate is used for seizure prophylaxis in severe preeclampsia.
- The only known cure of preeclampsia is delivery of the placenta. Early fetal delivery (based on totality of the case features, often by 37 weeks gestation) is the standard of care.
- Preeclampsia is associated with preterm birth and low birth weight babies.

Physiology Correlation. Intermediate trophoblast is an extravillous mononuclear cell that arises from cytotrophoblast and is important for placental implantation. It invades maternal spiral arteries early in the first trimester of pregnancy. The intermediate trophoblast also produces hormones that alter maternal physiology. Human placental lactogen (also produced by the syncytiotrophoblast) plays a role in maternal glucose metabolism; it increases the mass of maternal pancreatic islets during pregnancy.

Pharmacology Correlation. Intramuscular or IV magnesium sulfate is used to prevent and treat seizures in women with severe preeclampsia. Magnesium blocks neuromuscular transmission and inhibits acetylcholine release. The drug is excreted in the kidney, and urine output is monitored during use. Women are also monitored closely during treatment for indications of magnesium toxicity, such as loss of the patellar reflex. A serious adverse effect of treatment is maternal respiratory depression. The drug crosses the placenta and can cause fetal hypotension and hypotonia.

Vignette 9

A 60-year-old woman undergoes a screening mammography. A small, spiculated mass with a radiolucent core is detected. A stereotactic core needle biopsy is then done, and the histologic diagnosis is radial scar. An excisional biopsy is performed to rule out invasive carcinoma.

Pathogenesis. **Tubular carcinoma** (TC) **of the breast** is very rare (<5% of all breast cancers). Risk factors for TC are similar to risk factors for invasive ductal carcinoma (now called invasive carcinoma of no special type in the current WHO breast tumor classification). Family history, genetic mutations, moderate alcohol consumption, and postmenopausal hormone therapy are some known risk factors.

Clinical Presentation. The age at diagnosis is slightly younger than that of ductal carcinoma. The tumors tend to be small, nonpalpable lesions detected in the breast periphery on screening mammography. About a fifth may be multicentric. The tumor is rare in men. As seen in vignette 9, needle biopsy may fail to identify areas of invasive cancer.

Diagnostic Studies.
- U/S: hypoechoic mass with ill-defined margins and posterior acoustic shadowing.
- Mammography: small, spiculated mass with or without calcification
- Microscopic examination of tissue from needle or excisional biopsy
- Hormone-receptor status: TC is usually ER/PR positive and HER2 negative

Morphologic Features.
- Gross examination of breast biopsy: small (≤2 cm) infiltrative mass with a stellate cut surface
- Microscopic examination: 90% of tumor must have the well-differentiated tubular histology
  - Angulated tubules with open lumina in a dense, cellular stroma
  - No preservation of the myoepithelial cell layer
  - Epithelial cells with mild cytologic atypia, apical snouts, and a low mitotic rate

Differential Diagnosis. Microscopic examination is required to distinguish TC from other benign and malignant breast disease. Radial scar/complex sclerosing lesion may have the appearance of cancer on mammography and a benign appearance on needle biopsy; when excised there may be microscopic foci of invasive TC or invasive carcinoma not otherwise specified. In sclerosing adenosis the myoepithelial layer is preserved. If the tumor has an admixture of lobular and tubular histology, 90% of the cancer must be tubular by microscopy for the tubular prognosis to apply.

Treatment and Outcomes.

- Breast-conserving surgery with or without adjuvant radiotherapy
- Less commonly chemotherapy and hormonal therapy depending on other factors such as large tumor size or lymph node involvement
- Survival rate is 97% at 10 years
- Lower incidence of lymph node involvement or recurrence than invasive breast carcinoma of no special type
- There is an increased risk of developing an invasive carcinoma with a poorer prognosis in the contralateral breast.

Physiology Correlation. Hormone-receptor status is a factor that is used to establish breast cancer prognosis and therapy. Estrogen-receptor alpha is encoded by *ESR1*, a gene on chromosome 6. Because estrogen-receptor alpha plays a major role in breast cancer carcinogenesis and progression, it is a treatment target. About 70% of breast cancers are hormone receptor-positive. Progesterone positivity is regulated by estrogen so most cancers that are estrogen receptor positive are also progesterone receptor positive. Women with hormone-receptor positivity have longer disease-free survival. Tubular carcinoma cells are generally positive for estrogen and progesterone receptors. Tumors that are initially responsive to anti-estrogen therapy that become anti-estrogen resistant are said to have acquired resistance. Loss of estrogen receptor alpha expression underlies acquired endocrine resistance.

Pharmacology Correlation. Tamoxifen is a selective estrogen receptor modulator (SERM) that is an antagonist in breast tissue and a partial agonist in the endometrium. It is used with estrogen-receptor-positive breast cancer to reduce the risk of recurrence. It is also used to prevent breast cancer in women who are at high risk for the disease. It can be administered orally and is typically used for years. Side effects include vasoactive symptoms (hot flashes), headaches, visual changes, and irregular menstrual cycles; the drug increases risk of thrombosis and endometrial carcinoma. Tamoxifen is metabolized in the liver by cytochrome P450. Factors limiting response to tamoxifen therapy for breast cancer include concurrent therapy with certain selective serotonin reuptake inhibitors, including paroxetine and fluoxetine. Individuals with variant forms of the gene *CYP2D6* have varying levels of function of the enzyme cytochrome P450 2D6, which metabolizes about a quarter of all pharmacological drugs. Clinical tests are available to evaluate this enzyme's function.

Vignette 10

A 32-year-old woman presents with complaints of a left breast mass. She stopped nursing her newborn 2 weeks ago due to intolerable nipple pain. She is concerned about cancer because her maternal grandmother had breast cancer. On physical exam erythema and induration are noted in the upper inner quadrant of her left breast.

Pathogenesis. **Mastitis** occurs in 10% of breastfeeding women. Obstruction of milk flow in a lactiferous duct and stasis allows bacterial growth. **Acute mastitis** (AM) is most often caused by *S. aureus*, but other pathogens include *Strep* species, *Mycobacterium tuberculosis* and *Candida albicans*. The risk is higher in women who have experienced nipple pain or fissures and those who aren't on a regular lactation schedule. The incidence is higher in mothers of infants with cleft lip or palate.

Clinical Presentation. Most cases of AM occur in lactating women before the infant reaches 3 months of age. Women present with symptoms due to local inflammation in the breast and with generalized complaints of fever, headache, and malaise. Patients, like the one in vignette 10, often mention a history of nipple pain with a subsequent cessation or curtailment of their lactation schedule. Mastitis is generally unilateral. On examination a segment of the breast is red and indurated.

Diagnostic Studies.
- Diagnosis is made based on clinical history and physical examination
- Culture is usually performed only if patient does not improve on antibiotic therapy

Morphologic Features.
- Gross examination: if abscess formation is present, there may be a surrounding fibrous scar in the breast parenchyma
- Microscopy: acute and chronic inflammatory infiltrate involving ducts and lobules

Differential Diagnosis. The differential includes breast carcinoma. Inflammatory carcinoma of the breast presents with breast warmth, erythema, edema, and skin dimpling. Carcinoma becomes a more serious consideration if symptoms do not resolve with treatment for mastitis. Paget disease of the breast also affects the nipple/areolar complex. It typically presents with eczematoid changes of the nipple in postmenopausal women who may lack an underlying palpable mass but who are found to have ductal carcinoma in situ or invasive carcinoma of the breast on histologic examination. *Candida* mastitis typically causes a stabbing pain during lactation and pinking of the areola.

Treatment and Outcomes.
- Improvement of breastfeeding technique and application of warm compresses to facilitate complete drainage during feeds.
- Antibiotics for *Staph. aureus* and other bacterial infections; antifungal drugs for *Candida.*
- Abscess formation can occur requiring needle drainage under U/S or surgical drainage.
- Fistulas can develop.
- The pain of mastitis is a common reason for breastfeeding discontinuation, but continued breastfeeding aids resolution.
- Mastitis increases the risk of vertical transmission of HIV.

Physiology Correlation. Estrogen is required for mammogenesis, prolactin is required for synthesis and secretion of milk, and oxytocin is required for milk letdown (galactokinesis). Prolactin is produced by the anterior pituitary; its levels are high during pregnancy. Estrogen and progesterone levels fall after parturition, and absent their inhibition, prolactin binds to breast epithelial cell receptors to stimulate the synthesis of milk proteins. Oxytocin is produced by the posterior pituitary. It is released as a result of the nipple stimulation of suckling and the mother's thoughts about the baby; dopamine inhibits its secretion. Oxytocin binds to receptors on myoepithelial cells of the breast causing the ejection of milk into lactiferous ducts. Milk pools in lactiferous sinuses until it exits nipple pores. Milk ejection reflex is a neuroendocrine reflex. High levels of prolactin inhibit GnRH secretion from the hypothalamus and subsequently cause anovulation and lactation amenorrhea.

Pharmacology Correlation. Pregnant and breastfeeding women sometimes require pharmacologic treatment. Pregnancy increases plasma volume and decreases plasma protein binding, thereby altering the volume of distribution of drugs; for that reason alternate dosing regimens for pregnancy are sometimes part of product labeling. Most drugs are excreted in breast milk; drugs cross the maternal capillary membrane most importantly by passive diffusion. Antibiotics move across biological membranes to a greater extent when maternal protein binding of the drug is low. Another variable is the half-life of the drug, ie, drugs with a longer half-life are more likely to accumulate in milk.

Breast and Female Reproductive

Test What You Have Learned

1. A 55-year-old woman undergoes digital mammogram, which identifies a 1.5 cm spiculated mass in the right breast. Core biopsy of the lesion shows malignant angulated tubules with open lumina in a dense, cellular stroma. After excision of the tumor, if histologic examination identifies the tumor as estrogen-receptor positive, which of the following medications would be most useful to increase the patient's disease-free interval?

    A. Carboplatin
    B. Clomiphene citrate
    C. Magnesium sulfate
    D. Methotrexate
    E. Progestin
    F. Tamoxifen

2. A woman gives birth to a baby girl. The newborn examination is notable for excessive skin in the neck area. Ultrasound of the neck demonstrates multiple fluid-filled spaces in the soft tissue. The pediatrician is concerned about the possibility of other congenital abnormalities, and so orders further studies. Cardiac MRI demonstrates a bicuspid aortic valve and coarctation of the aorta. Which of the following complications would this infant be most likely to develop at age 7?

    A. Erythema nodosum
    B. Fistula formation
    C. Gonadoblastoma
    D. Hemorrhagic stroke
    E. Intrabdominal adhesion formation
    F. Uterine perforation

3. A 46-year-old woman with irregular menstrual periods undergoes uterine ultrasound at her gynecologist's office. The procedure reveals an increased thickness of her endometrial stripe. Endometrial curettage demonstrates an increased volume of endometrial tissue and an increased ratio of glands to stroma. Curettage reveals no atypia. This patient's uterine condition is most likely related to which of the following?

    A. Loss of PTEN gene

    B. HLA-B5+

    C. Serum CA125

    D. SHOX gene loss

    E. TP53 mutation

    F. Triploidy

4. A 37-year-old woman consults a clinic about infertility. She complains that her menstrual periods are irregular. Physical examination is notable for coarse hair on her chin and truncal obesity. Lab studies demonstrate increased ratio of LH/FSH. Which of the following medications would be the initial drug of choice?

    A. Carboplatin

    B. Clomiphene

    C. Metformin

    D. Methotrexate

    E. Oxytocin

5. A 47-year-old woman presents to the emergency room with a 2-week history of nausea and vomiting with accompanying excessive salivation and weakness. The patient is afebrile. A thorough review of symptoms does not suggest primary gastrointestinal, renal, or central nervous system disease. Obstetric ultrasonography demonstrates a "snowstorm" pattern in the uterus. Evacuation of the uterine contents would most likely demonstrate which of the following?

    A. Biphasic pattern of atypical syncytiotrophoblast and cytotrophoblast with no chorionic villi present

    B. Diffuse villous edema with circumferential trophoblastic proliferation

    C. Increased ratio of normal appearing endometrial glands to stroma

    D. Placental tissue with small villi and villous syncytial knots

    E. Some edematous villi with focal trophoblastic proliferation

Answers: 1. (F), 2. (C), 3. (A), 4. (B), 5. (B)

Vignette Diagnoses

Chapter 1: Hematopoietic and Lymphoreticular System

Vignette 1. 22q11.2 deletion syndrome

Vignette 2. Thymoma

Vignette 3. G6PD deficiency

Vignette 4. Cutaneous mastocytosis

Vignette 5. Lymphoblastic lymphoma

Vignette 6. Acute myelogenous leukemia

Vignette 7. Myelodysplastic syndrome

Vignette 8. Immune thrombocytopenic purpura

Vignette 9. Polycythemia as a paraneoplastic syndrome in renal cell carcinoma

Vignette 10. Cat-scratch disease

Chapter 2: Nervous System and Special Senses

Vignette 1. Fetal alcohol syndrome

Vignette 2. Subdural hematoma

Vignette 3. Guillain-Barré

Vignette 4. Huntington disease

Vignette 5. Basilar artery thrombosis

Vignette 6. Creutzfeldt-Jacob disease (CJD)

Vignette 7. Meningioma

Vignette 8. Toxoplasma encephalitis

Vignette 9. Ménière's disease

Vignette 10. Postural orthostatic tachycardia syndrome

Chapter 3: Musculoskeletal System

Vignette 1. Osteogenesis imperfecta

Vignette 2. Lyme disease

Vignette 3. Gout

Chapter 6: Respiratory System

Vignette 1. Neonatal respiratory distress syndrome

Vignette 2. Cryptogenic organizing pneumonia (COP)

Vignette 3. Idiopathic pulmonary fibrosis

Vignette 4. Hypersensitivity pneumonitis

Vignette 5. Cystic fibrosis

Vignette 6. Typical carcinoid

Vignette 7. Tuberculosis

Vignette 8. Tension pneumothorax

Vignette 9. Malignant pleural mesothelioma

Vignette 10. Pulmonary hypertension

Chapter 7: Gastrointestinal System

Vignette 1. Barrett esophagus

Vignette 2. Autoimmune atrophic gastritis

Vignette 3. Gastric lymphoma

Vignette 4. Typhoid fever

Vignette 5. Pseudomembranous colitis

Vignette 6. Crohn disease

Vignette 7. Wilson disease

Vignette 8. Primary sclerosing cholangitis

Vignette 9. Hirschsprung disease

Vignette 10. Necrotizing enterocolitis

Chapter 8: Renal and Urinary System

Vignette 1. Wilms tumor

Vignette 2. Hemolytic uremic syndrome (HUS)

Vignette 3. Minimal change disease

Vignette 4. Systemic lupus erythematosus

Vignette 5. Amyloidosis

Vignette 6. Chronic obstructive pyelonephritis

Vignette 7. Nephrotoxic acute tubular injury from organic solvent exposure